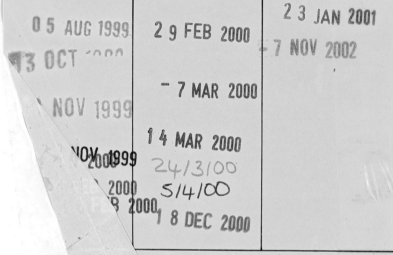

Stress Management in Primary Care

Kenneth Hambly and Alice Jane Muir

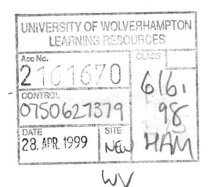
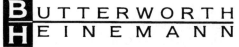
BUTTERWORTH
HEINEMANN

Butterworth-Heinemann
Linacre House, Jordan Hill, Oxford OX2 8DP
A division of Reed Educational and Professional Publishing Ltd

$\mathcal{R}$ A member of the Reed Elsevier plc group

OXFORD   BOSTON   JOHANNESBURG
MELBOURNE   NEW DELHI   SINGAPORE

First published 1997

British Library Cataloguing in Publication Data

A catalogue record for this book is available from the British Library

Library of Congress Cataloguing in Publication Data

A catalogue record for this book is available from the Library of Congress

ISBN 0 7506 2737 9

Typeset by E & M Graphics, Midsomer Norton, Bath
Printed and bound in Great Britain by Biddles Ltd, Guildford and King's Lynn

Contents

Introduction

Doctors and psychologists do not always speak the same language. This is unfortunate because we often share the same interests, particularly if the doctor is in general practice where so many patients suffer from psychological problems such as stress. When we, the authors of this book (Ken Hambly, a GP in a semi-rural practice in Ayrshire, and Alice Muir, a trainer and psychologist), started the Stewarton Stress Management Project, we had to learn to talk to each other and understand each other. Initially, that was not easy.

We had an interest in common in the treatment of stress. Ken Hambly has written for the medical profession for many years and has also written six books on related topics for the lay public. Alice Muir had been involved in stress management and other training since the early 1980s, within adult education and the voluntary sector, and had compiled a wide range of resources and booklets for this purpose. We thus had a common interest in writing and communication and so it was not surprising that, as the project developed, we began to think about writing a book about stress management.

We come from different academic backgrounds, so we approached the subject of stress from divergent perspectives. Our common purpose was in constructing an accessible stress management clinic, which would be run by practice nurses or other paramedical staff in any general practice. We had generous funding from the Ayrshire and Arran Health Board and the Scottish Office to help us to achieve this end. We found that we had a lot more in common than this objective and that each of us had expanded the other's understanding of the problems of stress and the difficulties in managing patients suffering from stress. We decided to put our ideas into print.

This book is therefore based on the fruits of our co-operation in the Stewarton Stress Management Project. It is intended to inform and assist other GPs, GP registrars, medical students and paramedical staff who may find themselves in the position of having to treat stressed patients. It is a practical text based on our experience, our successes and failures, and our hopes for the future of the important subject of stress management in primary care.

It is hoped that our readers will be able to improve their skills in this area of practice and to communicate these skills to others. They may wish to seek training for ancillary staff so that they will be able to set up a service for stressed patients within their practice and generally to improve the management of this increasingly important group. These patients now expect such treatment, which we feel should be within the compass of every general practice to provide.

It is thus the intention of this book to improve the management of stress related disorders by doctors, with particular reference to general practice in its broader sense, where the primary care team can be involved in all aspects of care. We hope that we have shown that doctors and psychologists can work well together, that their ideas and approaches are compatible, and that at the end of the day we do speak the same language.

We end with a chapter on the stress experienced by GPs themselves because of the nature of their occupation, and how this problem can be combated and managed. For some this may be the most important chapter of all and we commend it to our readers. It is our hope that this is a book from which all can benefit – students, patients, ancillary staff and doctors – because it expresses in simple accessible language our practical experience of the problems of stress management.

We acknowledge the help and support of Drew Walker of the Ayrshire and Arran Health Board, and of Ann Marie Lynch and Marion Welsh, the practice nurses in the Stewarton practice, who had the difficult task of putting the Stewarton 'Stresswise' project into effect.

Part One
Stress in Context

1

An overview   Symptoms!

Why concern ourselves about stress? Surely we have enough to worry about without taking on the role of stress counsellor? Unfortunately, a doctor cannot ignore stress. Stress is a problem, and it contributes a great deal to the morbidity in our community. We ignore it at our peril. It is an increasingly important topic in primary care and anyone who reads the lay press cannot fail to have an awareness of the problems it produces. Despite this, it is almost impossible to find a simple unifying definition of stress. We know what we mean, or at least we think we know what we mean, but it is difficult to pin down the real nature of stress as a disease entity. How do you define stress? Try it, and you will see how difficult it is.

Stress: a definition

It must be possible to arrive at a precise definition of stress so that at least we know what we are talking about when we discuss stress management. The word stress is used loosely to describe several concepts. Overwork, debt or relationship problems could all be described as a form of stress, but what an individual feels or experiences in such situations is also described as stress. This is clearly a confusing basis from which to begin, so, for the purposes of this book, stress will be taken to refer to people's experience of stress rather than the situation in which they find themselves. Now at least we know what we mean by stress.

We are talking about stress as a problem, but, to add to the confusion, the experience of some stress is not necessarily a bad thing. We all need some stress or challenge in our lives in order to perform at our best, or rather, there is an optimum level of autonomic arousal at which we perform tasks best; below this, or above it, we perform less well. Arousal is part of our biological make-up, and it is necessary if we are to prepare ourselves physically to cope with whatever situation we will experience. In dealing with stress as a medical condition we are probably really dealing with a patient who has a maladaptively high level of autonomic arousal or who has moved from an anabolic to a catabolic physiological milieu. We can add that concept to our definition of stress.

The problem is that an ability to produce high levels of arousal evolved in prehistoric human beings as a means of dealing with threatening or endangering situations, largely of a physical nature. This arousal was usually only required over relatively short periods of time, a few minutes or hours perhaps. Still higher levels could act over even shorter periods of time to allow our ancestors either to fight or to flee, as all medical students know. This arousal prepared our ancestors for a physical response and was useful and adaptive, anabolic and essentially sympathetic adrenomedullary. So much for the physiology of stress.

However, in our modern world, although a short burst of appropriately high arousal can be helpful, situations such as debt or overwork can provoke this response continually for days, months or even years. Added to this, the physiological response to these situations prepares us for a physical reaction, but, in today's world, there is seldom an outlet for that reaction. This response is neither useful nor adaptive, and the individual may become over-reactive, producing ever higher levels of arousal in response to new or continuing situations. High arousal can continue long after the situation provoking it has disappeared; if this happens, the individual response to stress becomes primarily pituitary adrenocortical and therefore catabolic.

Another aspect of stress is that it can be acute in that there may be unhelpfully high levels of arousal occurring only in response to short-lived situations. Alternatively, or in addition, it may be chronic in that unhelpfully high levels of arousal continue to be maintained during and sometimes after a long-term situation. In either case, the result is the same. With no outlet for this arousal, the affected person will experience a range of unpleasant physical, psychological and behavioural symptoms that are commonly described and experienced as stress. That is another way of thinking about stress. Let us try for a unifying definition.

For the purpose of this book, stress is defined as follows: *Stress is a condition in which there is a maladaptively high level of adrenergic arousal, which may be acute and/or chronic, resulting in a range of unpleasant physical, psychological and behavioural problems.*

This would seem to be a more practical definition of stress than the traditional one, which defines anything that raises an organism's adrenocorticotrophic hormone (ACTH) level as being a source of stress, and defines the stress response as being an elevation of ACTH and glucocorticoid concentrations. The latter definition is more appropriate for research purposes, but here we are dealing with practicalities.

The symptoms

Stressed patients experience symptoms. It is the onset of these symptoms that brings them to the doctor's surgery, and it is these symptoms that create the dilemma for the GP. Treating stress-induced symptoms is not traditionally part of a GP's training and the treatment options available are not those usually used by GPs in their daily surgeries, yet stressed patients continue to present and continue to demand treatment. GPs understand well the physiological rationale for the patient's complaints, but the logical diagnosis and treatment of stress-related problems is a more elusive topic.

A patient may present in the consulting room complaining that he or she is stressed, or the patient may describe symptoms or feelings that may be frightening or disturbing, but which are not initially attributed to stress. Patients may deny stress, even to themselves, preferring to present a physical problem. As with every presenting complaint, a good history will clarify the situation and greatly contribute to patient management. The patient may, for example, describe one of the physical symptoms listed below:

- Headaches;
- Indigestion;
- Churning stomach;
- Palpitations;
- Difficulty in taking a deep breath;
- Difficulty with swallowing;
- Tingling of the peripheries;
- Nausea;
- Fatigue;
- Aches and pains;
- Muscle twitches;
- Sweating;
- Muscle tension;
- Weight gain or loss;
- Trembling;
- Dry mouth;
- Insomnia;
- Poor balance;
- Light-headedness;
- Hyperventilation.

Such physical symptoms are unlikely to occur in isolation and there will usually be an overlay of psychological problems, which can be more frightening. The patient may experience attacks of panic or other symptoms that have both a physical and a psychological component. Psychological symptoms may even predominate and be freely voluntered by the patient, or they may be admitted on further questioning. Symptoms with a psychological contribution are:

- Anxiety;
- Worry;
- Depression;
- Panic attacks;
- Negative outlook;
- Hopelessness;
- Fearfulness;
- Gloomy thoughts;
- Withdrawal;
- Feelings of unreality;
- Feelings of depersonalization;
- Feeling unable to cope.

There is a further element to stress-related problems, which may not always be considered by the GP. Stress, like many other medical conditions, can change behaviour. These behavioural changes may be of great importance to the patient, whose marriage, job or career, or social life can be threatened. A list of common behavioural problems is given below:

- Restlessness;
- Agitation;
- Making mistakes;
- Forgetfulness;
- Poor concentration;
- Violent outbursts;
- Change in usual behaviour;
- Pacing;
- Hand-wringing;
- Indecision;
- Anger;
- Shouting;
- Irritability;

- Aggression;
- Eating too much or too little;
- Inability to cope;
- Increased substance use.

The history of a stress-related condition

Stress may begin as a trivial or manageable condition, as an annoyance or an inconvenience. Everyone has experienced stress and everyone has some understanding of what it can be like. In industry and business, as in sport, people are expected to be able to manage stress, and most people can do so, up to a point. Some people are better at managing stress than others, but everyone has a point beyond which they cannot continue to manage it without experiencing problems. These problems may be physical, psychological or behavioural, but they have an effect on the patient's life and this effect can be profound and disturbing.

The longer the stress continues, the more serious the effects can become. A patient may become exhausted, chronically agitated and unable to sleep. This can lead to a complete inability to cope and withdrawal from the day-to-day routine, or to a state of anxiety or clinical depression, and even the risk of suicide. There is also evidence to suggest that stress may play a part in causing a number of common physical and psychological conditions such as heart disease, hypertension, insomnia, muscle pains, peptic ulcers, irritable bowel syndrome, fatigue, panic disorder, phobias and obsessions.

In addition to this, many physical conditions are made worse by stress, including asthma, psoriasis, eczema, migraine and numerous other illnesses. Stress can affect the immune system, although the sequelae of this are unclear. Advice on how to manage stress is therefore of very great and increasing importance in general practice. We therefore have to know about it; we have to understand it; we have to be able to treat it.

The extent of the problem

There is a very real feeling in the general community that stress itself is on the increase. GPs would undoubtedly concur and the statistics would seem to bear this out. Acute stress disorders are thought to account for as many as 10 per cent of cases of mental illness identified by GPs, and time off work due to stress-related illness is estimated to have increased fivefold between the 1950s and the 1990s.

Every working day, an estimated 270 000 people in England and Wales take time off work because of stress-related mental illness. This is clearly a major problem, bearing in mind that the everyday stress-induced symptoms such as insomnia, tension headache, neck pain and low-grade anxiety may never reach the statistical records. All of this is reflected in the number of patients presenting at GPs' surgeries seeking help. So what help is available? What can the besieged GP do? Fortunately, a range of effective and practical techniques is available for dealing with this time-consuming and increasingly large group of patients.

Managing stress

Stress management may be strange territory for the GP, but the techniques used are actually relatively inexpensive and straightforward. Some may be well known to the GP and some may not. In general, they are not techniques that the GP will use routinely in everyday practice. The techniques are based on common-sense principles and can be learned and applied. Patients are receptive to these approaches and willing to try them, and are always grateful for the help they receive.

Before coming to see a GP, patients will often have made matters worse by using coping strategies that seem like the right thing to do, but actually compound the problem. They may well not be aware that their problem is stress, so they may be working longer hours, taking fewer breaks, sleeping less, eating irregularly, smoking, overeating or drinking too much alcohol or coffee, all of which increase the problem. They need rational treatment, but what treatment?

There is always going to be a role for drugs in coping with stress, if they are used correctly, especially in the short-term, but drugs are of limited use and there has to be another answer that encourages patients to manage their own condition in order to obtain long-term benefit. What else can patients do to help themselves? What practical steps can be taken to manage stress?

A history of stress management techniques

Stress management itself dates back to the First World War, during which many soldiers suffered from 'shell shock'. This was then assumed to be a neurological dysfunction resulting from brain damage caused by the sound of exploding shells. However, during the Second World War, this condition came to be thought of as an emotional breakdown caused by the 'stress' of combat, and was described as 'battle fatigue' or 'war neurosis'. After 1945, there was a growing realization that many situations in everyday life could also provoke similar effects to battle fatigue. This, teamed with an interest by the military in training men to manage stress, gave rise to the development of stress management.

More recently, increasing attention has been paid to the true nature of battle fatigue, now termed post-traumatic stress syndrome, which is now recognized as occuring not just in response to battle but to a wide range of traumatic events.

The techniques used

In general terms, the physical nature of acute stress is the increase in autonomic arousal, so the techniques used in treating it are in the main those that reduce this autonomic arousal. These methods allow the patient to begin to regain control of his or her autonomic nervous system and are essentially logical and straightforward. They are based on a range of well tried behavioural and psychological techniques.

Relaxation exercises

If a muscle is consciously tensed and then released, it will relax. If muscle groups are tensed and relaxed systematically, the patient will physically relax.

Breathing exercises

Chronic disorders of respiration play an important part in the generation and maintenance of the physical symptoms found in stressed patients. Simple breathing exercises can restore normal breathing patterns and reduce the severity of the patient's symptoms.

Lifestyle changes

It is usually impossible or inadvisable for a patient to suddenly effect major changes in his or her lifestyle. The GP cannot solve financial problems or workplace problems or save a failing marriage, no matter how desirable this might be, but small changes can have a major effect. Taking regular breaks and more exercise will be of advantage. The control of smoking and alcohol use can also help, as can advice about coffee consumption and healthy eating.

Sorting out priorities

Patients may feel that their lives are in a mess and that they cannot cope. Coping strategies such as sorting out priorities and seeking social support can be taught.

Reducing stress

In an ideal world, it would be important to do something about the causes of the patient's stress. This may not be possible, but sometimes a patient can make personal decisions that will help to resolve the problem.

The General Practitioner and stress management

GPs in the UK have an average of seven and a half minutes in which to: welcome a patient; engage with the patient and obtain a history; examine the patient, make a diagnosis and agree that diagnosis; and then initiate treatment, before dismissing that patient and calling the next. How this is achieved is sometimes difficult to explain to those not involved in the process, but it is certainly a highly skilled and under-valued exercise. It is within this framework that the doctor must con-template the diagnosing and treating of stress-related disorders. Even if the doctor has all the skill and expertise available, there will always be the constraints of time.

GPs have certain advantages over other doctors and health care workers. Patients' expectations are limited by their understanding and acceptance of the system and they are prepared to work within its limitations. This is something rarely understood by patients from abroad. The GP will know the patient and the family and will often have a detailed knowledge of the circumstances related to the visit. The doctor can also ask the patient to return for further investigation and treatment, and, on occasions, there may be the flexibility to extend the duration of the appointment.

The benefits to the GP in treating stress-related problems are con-siderable. Apart from the professional satisfaction of managing the condition well, the doctor may be able to reduce the number of visits a frequent attender will make, and the treatment of many difficult and time-consuming disorders will be rendered feasible, thus increasing patient satisfaction. The GP, therefore, can make major gains.

Apart from these benefits, the doctor has no option but to treat stress-related disorders because they present in the surgery. It is possible to treat most of these presentations symptomatically or to prevaricate without really addressing the problem, but the patient is there and the patient is demanding treatment. As with any condition the GP sees, a diagnosis is required and so is the initiation of some kind of treatment. The doctor must be able to respond. Of course, all doctors do respond in their own way, but what is being advocated here is a more logical and rational approach to the condition.

Stages of management

Initial management must be by the GP because the patient has chosen to attend the surgery. Stressed patients seek urgent treatment and deserve urgent treatment because they will be at the end of their tether. Some form of stress management will therefore be required at the first visit. What happens after the first consultation is a matter of choice for the GP. Various options are available, depending on the confidence and interest of the doctor and the severity of the patient's problem. The more likely options are as follows:

- The doctor may continue management using printed hand-outs or tapes.
- Referral to a clinical psychologist, community psychiatric nurse or counsellor may be appropriate.
- Self-help groups or adult education classes may be available, to which the patient can be referred.
- The doctor may decide to initiate a stress management clinic run under his or her direction by health care professionals, thus keeping treatment within the practice.

It is possible to treat a patient in stages, beginning with simple supportive techniques with the option of referring later. Many patients will respond well to empathetic treatment by the doctor, who may use his or her own experience, together with appropriate hand-outs or tapes. Patients who do not respond may require referral for more expert treatment.

Often stress will be part of a differential diagnosis and some investigation will be necessary. Dealing with the actual cause of the patient's difficulty can be deferred and the definitive diagnosis arrived at by degrees. Most GPs will be familiar with this approach and have considerable expertise in its execution.

Who suffers from stress and why?

Anyone can suffer from stress. Socially deprived groups are more likely to be exposed to stressful life events than those who are more affluent. Women also seem to be more at risk than men, and the age group of 35–45 years is the most seriously affected. Figure 1.1 shows the results of a recent study carried out by the General Practice Administration Scheme (Scotland) (GPASS) Data Evaluation Project at the Department of General Practice, University of Aberdeen, which recorded the diagnoses of over 100 000 patients attending 35 practices over a two-year period ending in 1995.

There is clearly a wide range of situations that can give rise to stress: unemployment, debt, relationship problems, single-handed caring for an elderly person or small children, difficult neighbours, illness, difficult teenagers, overwork, loneliness, deprivation, crime or bereavement; the list could go on and on. Even the daily hassles typical of modern living can become stressful and in time produce symptoms. Workplace stress is also common in our harsh economic climate, with increasing pressure upon employees to perform above their abilities and staff cuts making jobs increasingly difficult.

There are also situations that will produce stress in one individual but

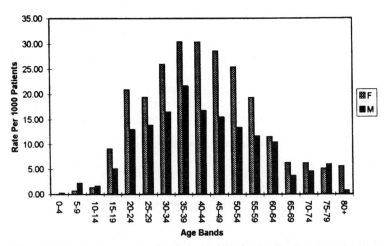

Age/Sex Distribution of Acute Reaction to Stress

Figure 1.1 Consultation rates per 1000 for acute stress reaction in men and women, from a sample of over 100 000 patients from 35 practices taken over two years, ending in 1995. (Reproduced by kind permission of the GPASS Data Evaluation Project, Department of General Practice, University of Aberdeen.)

not in another. Childlessness, for example, may cause acute stress in many couples, but, in others, this is their considered choice. City driving is a major problem to many, but an ordinary task to others. Stress is the result of interaction between the person and the situation in which they find themselves. This interaction will decide whether or not that situation is perceived as a threat and so will produce stress. Many situations experienced by one person as provoking acute stress may be experienced by another as a challenge, or even as an everyday event. Particular situations can therefore provoke stress in some people but not in others, depending on people's personalities and experiences of life. Moreover, some people have a nervous system that is more labile, and therefore more likely to become easily aroused.

Therefore, in most day-to-day situations, how individuals appraise and then deal with situations largely determines whether or not they will experience stress; this is very much down to constitution, personality and previous experience.

An approach to the stressed patient

A doctor can adequately treat a condition only if he or she is comfortable with the diagnosis and familiar with the treatment options. This applies to any medical condition, but some conditions are more straightforward than others and have fewer therapeutic options. A GP may feel that stress is not his or her problem, that it is not a medical condition at all, but increasingly patients will present with stress-related conditions and inevitably it will be a problem the doctor has to be able to manage. Clinical psychologists, community psychiatric nurses and counsellors may be qualified to provide treatment, but it is the doctor to whom the patient comes first and who must make the diagnosis. For the distressed patient, it is the doctor who must respond and initiate treatment.

The non-specific nature of stress can also cause difficulties and may appear to defy a unified approach, so that the GP is less than comfortable in making the diagnosis. Stress in others can even seem threatening to GPs themselves. The patient is stressed; what do I do now? What resources do I have, both personal and practical? This book aims to answer such questions and provide information and resources that will make diagnosis and treatment much more straightforward.

Diagnosis and treatment

Both diagnosis and treatment depend upon good consultation techniques; such skills can be practised and improved. Empathy and reassurance and a positive response to the presenting complaint are as always appropriate, and, for the confused, frightened or demoralized stressed patient, the right attitude can be life-saving. A stressed patient successfully treated will always be the most grateful patient of the day.

Even if the diagnosis is not initially obvious, it is not necessarily a diagnosis of exclusion in every case. Good history-taking can establish the diagnosis to the satisfaction of both the doctor and the patient, but, when there is doubt, appropriate investigations or referrals may be necessary as in any other medical condition. Although stress may seem to produce a rag-bag of symptoms and problems, there are many symptoms that are common to all stressed patients and for which standard techniques can be used in treatment.

Often, the establishment of the diagnosis is sufficient to provide considerable relief to a patient who has had difficulty in admitting to a stress-related disorder, or who may have come in the belief that they are suffering from a major physical illness. Relieved patients may sometimes admit that they thought they were going mad. The stressed patient may seem well protected and appear to resist the diagnosis, but, once it is made, the flood gates can open and the problem may be unexpectedly aired.

The role of the General Practitioner

Summoning up the appropriate emotional response to the stressed patient is not easy. It may depend upon how the doctor feels and upon what time of the day or week it is. It is the particular skill of GPs that they can deal in quick succession with the child with a sore throat, the patient with a possible malignant condition, and the stressed individual in consecutive short appointments of a few minutes' duration. No one should underestimate the skill this involves. Engaging with a stressed patient and, just as importantly, disengaging again in the space of a short appointment, is extremely demanding. It requires skill, professionalism and considerable personal resources.

Treating stress is something the doctor must want to do. It is possible to avoid making the diagnosis, to treat the patient symptomatically or to offer a quick prescription, but treating stress is a challenge, which, if faced, can bring its own rewards. Frequent attenders can become self-sufficient and difficult patients can change to being co-operative and manageable. Treating stress allows the doctor to adopt effective skills and techniques developed over decades by psychologists and others. Cultivating new personal skills is always a challenge and a source of satisfaction. As already mentioned, the stressed patient successfully treated will always be both relieved and grateful.

Stress and the General Practitioner

Any consideration of the problems of stress in general practice would be incomplete if it did not address the stressful nature of general practice itself. The stress of being exposed daily to depressed, terminally ill or chronically sick patients is often quoted as a cause of stress, but a more potent cause is the constantly increasing workload and the difficulty of time management in an unpredictable profession.

Increased patient expectations and patient demands that cannot be met have been identified as a cause of stress, but the most potent reason why GPs experience stress is the requirement to work out of hours and be available to treat anything from the infant who 'just won't settle' to the patient with a coronary thrombosis or intracranial haemorrhage. Long hours and sleep deprivation are a prescription for stress and it is important that GPs should take active steps to protect themselves against it.

In conclusion

Stress has not just recently been invented; neither has it just been discovered. Medical practitioners, psychologists and others have described it and advocated methods of treating it for decades, but it has been neglected as a medical condition by mainstream clinical practice. GPs treat it empirically, often very well, but our medical schools still tend to ignore conditions that cannot be palpated, excised or medicated. The treatment methods appropriate to the management of stress are well known and well described, and they work. Time spent in considering them is time well spent, and will produce benefits for the doctor both in terms of the quality of medical care and the quality of patient satisfaction.

Summary

- Stress is defined here as the patient's experience of high autonomic arousal for which there is no outlet in the modern world.
- Stress therefore produces a wide range of physical, psychological and behavioural symptoms.
- Anyone from any background can become stressed, but this is more likely in women, particularly those who are socially or economically deprived.
- Stress plays a part in causing a range of physiological conditions.

- Chronic stress can also lead to other more serious psychological and physiological conditions.
- Stress is very common and appears to be on the increase.
- A range of straightforward and effective techniques can be used for managing stress.
- These can be made available to the patient in a number of ways.
- The stressed patient has a strong emotional overlay.
- Appropriate consultation skills are important in dealing with the stressed patient.
- GP stress must also be addressed.

2

Life stress and workplace stress

Stress today

We live in a world in which change is both rapid and endemic. There is little that is predictable and within our control, and people no longer know what to expect out of life. Gone is the 'job for life', to be replaced by the fixed-term contract, or worse, unemployment. With increasing equality of the sexes, the old certainties of role and expectations from life, however unsatisfactory these were, have also gone. With increasing secularity, people have less commitment and meaning to their lives. We live in the so called 'global village', where news travels as fast as light, and we are faced daily with the war, tragedy and trauma of others in our living rooms. In contrast, we may not even know the person who lives next door to us. Gone are the days of leaving doors unlocked, and having granny and auntie within a street or two. Many people today are entirely ruled by the clock, with more and more to be squeezed into less and less time, both at work and at home. Material possessions, success and ability to cope are prized in today's world. All of this is a heavy burden for a body designed for the Stone Age.

It is a difficult exercise to estimate just how many people suffer the effects of stress. As we have seen, stress can produce a wide range of physical, psychological and behavioural symptoms, many of which go unrecorded in terms of stress statistics. Only patients diagnosed as clearly experiencing 'acute stress disorder' are recorded as such.

Furthermore, Rachel Jenkins, of the Department of Health, asserted at a CBI conference in 1992 that the most common psychological illnesses are depression and anxiety, and that these are mostly caused by environmental stresses. Also, as has already been mentioned, anxiety can lead to more serious conditions such as phobias, panic attacks and obsessions. Indeed, as doctors are aware, mental health problems constitute up to 40 per cent of all symptoms reported to them.

Taking all these complicating factors into account the following statistics will merely confirm the extent of the problem:

- In 1991, working days lost through stress and anxiety cost UK industry £4100 million.

- In the course of a year, 12 million adults consulting their GPs have mental health problems; of these, 80 per cent suffer from anxiety and depressive states.
- Up to 10 per cent of the population suffer from anxiety or depression at any one time.
- The lifetime prevalence of phobias is 13 per cent.
- In a 1985 study, 36 per cent of the general population reported one or more panic attacks in the past year, with 17 per cent having had an attack in the previous month.
- 'In 1991, GPs issued 19 million prescriptions for benzodiazepine sedatives, tranquillisers and hypnotics at a cost to the NHS of aproximately £19 million' (MIND, 1995).
- According to MIND and the World Health Organization, social problems producing family stress are crucial factors in suicide risk.
- Every two hours in the UK, someone commits suicide.

The stress equation

In order to explain the varied and cumulative nature of stress, Professor Cary Cooper and his colleagues (1988) have developed and described their 'stress equation' as follows:

$$\text{Life stress} + \text{Work stress} + \text{Individual vulnerability} = \text{Stress symptoms/outcomes}$$

This neatly encapsulates all the components that can contribute to an individual's experience of stress and demonstrates its multifaceted nature. All stress, from whatever source, simply aggregates to build up the overall picture, which is unique to the individual. These three components will be considered in detail in this chapter and in Chapter 3.

It is also worth noting at this point that this equation is not the whole story. There is also a multiplier effect at work here, whereby stress in one area of life can put pressure on another area, thus escalating the whole problem. If someone is having difficulty with his or her boss, this will probably spill over into the home and family life, increasing stress there too. However, it is still a useful model to use to help us to steer our way through a multifaceted phenomenon.

Are we more stressed today?

Each period of human history has produced its own distinctive crop of plagues, wars, pestilences and famines. Should there not therefore be less stress nowadays instead of more, with relatively few of such dreadful and life-threatening problems to face? The simple answer is no, we are actually more at the mercy of stress today for several reasons.

First, in the past, society was less complex, and the episodes of stress were in the main few and far between, compared with the chronic stress of today's sophisticated world. Even in recent times, during two world wars, people had a sense of being part of one nation with everyone on the same side, pulling together and supporting one another. This ameliorated considerably the effects of a time of great stress. Secondly, we are today very much ruled by the clock; unrelenting time pressure has been placed upon many of us. A few centuries ago, all that mattered was that it was mid-afternoon, now we need to know that it is exactly 3.25 p.m., and we still have two meetings to fit in, or there are still 10 patients in the waiting room. Lastly, life today is ever-changing, and the rate of change is on the increase. We constantly have to make readjustments to our lives; all of these changes produce another small injection of arousal and stress.

Every historical period and every society has its own idea of what life and human nature is all about. Current western society emphasizes the importance of the successful, independent and autonomous individual, exercising choice and making decisions in a materialistic world. This automatically places continuous stress on people to strive for material success: the rat race, in other words. This emphasis on the successful individual is by no means a universal concept. Other societies do not share this view of life. Historical and cross-cultural studies suggest that, in other cultures, the community or society itself may be more important, or individuals and their society can be blurred into one. The Javanese and Balinese, for example, believe that all personal expression is impolite and vulgar. Whilst not suggesting that everyone moves to Bali or Java to escape stress, we must recognize that stress is very much an outcome of the nature of late-twentieth-century life in western society.

It is with this backdrop that we now look at the stresses of life in the UK today. Individual vulnerability to stress will be covered in the next chapter, but we turn now to focus on life and workplace stresses. All doctors are unhappily familiar with the wide-ranging social and economic problems that affect their patients. Sadly, the traumas of life are laid painfully bare to them on a daily basis. This chapter aims to provide a deeper and broader insight into a range of the stresses of life and their unhappy outcomes.

Life stresses

Raising a family

Parents today find it increasingly difficult to know how best to raise their children. They fear getting it wrong, and they fear what may happen to their children if they do. They are bombarded with magazine articles and discussion programmes advocating this or that method of parenting, and are often the target of blame when things go wrong. Today's parents have a succession of problems to deal with which their parents could not even have imagined, and there is no firm agreement on how these should be tackled. The youngest of children are exposed to drugs, with dealers around every corner. No longer can children walk unaccompanied to evening activities such as Brownies or Scouts. Statistics do not bear out an increased risk to children on the streets from a malevolent stranger, but parents still fear it, because of media treatment of the subject. Violent and sexually explicit material is easily available to children, and parents do not know how to deal with this. Even the so-called experts cannot make up their minds, so what are parents expected to do? What about the effect on young minds of endless hours playing computer games? The jury is still out on that one too.

Parents now talk about 'peer group pressure' and 'sibling rivalry' in the way that the previous generation of parents used to talk about whether or not to let their sons out of short trousers, or to allow their daughters to wear nylons.

Change is outstripping society's ability to make up its mind about new activities and experiences, leaving parents totally at sea. Yet, according to Relate, if parents cannot communicate positively and consistently with their children, there will be a host of negative outcomes for these children, including depression, drug and alcohol use, and criminality.

As if all this was not bad enough, the break-up of old relationships and the forming of new ones has produced still other new situations with which parents must cope. How do you deal with lone parenthood, two children with different fathers, second families or step-children? Relate has predicted that by the year 2000, 3 million children and young people will be growing up in a step-family.

These desperate difficulties are often combined with struggling to amalgamate family with work, in order to make ends meet or to keep up in an increasingly materialistic society. The feminist movement of the 1960s has done little to liberate women. Most now find that they are expected both to work and to have a family. Relate reports that, even in families in which both partners work full-time, the woman continues to shoulder the main reponsibility for the home.

We now have an uneasy picture of parenthood, which includes constant change teamed with overwork, unpredictability and a feeling of a lack of control. These are all factors that increase vulnerabilty to stress, as we shall see later.

Case history 2.1

Margaret comes into the surgery a little too briskly, and sits down uneasily. She looks agitated, and desperate for a cigarette, as she smokes 40 a day, though she insists she is trying to give up. 'I'm living on my nerves doctor', she says. 'I've got constant headaches, and I can't eat. Look at me, I'm wasting away.' She continues almost without taking a breath, 'It's these two boys of mine. They fight all the time, and the oldest one has just been suspended from school for giving cheek to teachers. I can't do anything with him, he just says what am I going to do about it. He's nearly six feet, and I'm five feet two. He won't listen to Robert, because he says he's not his real dad, and he says Jamie is our favourite because Robert is his real dad.'

Personal relationships

Whatever one's views on the subject, the old presumption and stability of a marriage made in heaven and expected to last for ever has most certainly disappeared:

- In 1991, only 25 per cent of households contained the traditional nuclear family.
- Since the 1970s, marriage rates in the UK have fallen by 16 per cent, whereas divorces have more than doubled.
- Cohabitation prior to marriage is now normal practice, and yet this actually increases the likelihood of a subsequent divorce.
- In 1992, there were 190 000 new petitions for divorce in England and Wales, the highest rate in Europe.
- The number of lone parents doubled between 1971 and 1991; 90 per cent of these are women. Only a third of lone parents have never been married.

The stress of parenting has already been described; and all to often on top of this is piled the appalling pain and stress of divorce and separation. There are also likely to be changes in lifestyle, home and financial status for both partners, which only add to the burden of stress. What we have here is a minefield of stresses for thousands of people, which can drift on and on for many years.

Violence and abuse in families

Gelles wrote in 1979 that, 'People are more likely to be hit, beat up, physically injured or even killed in their own homes by another family member than anywhere else, and by anyone else, in our society.'

Unlike some of the life stresses already discussed, domestic violence is not new; it goes back for many centuries. It also occurs in all cultures, and happens to women from all walks of life. Doctors will already be fully acquainted with the problem because they treat its victims, but here is some information from Relate and Women's Aid which paints a poignant and perhaps wider picture:

- One half to one-third of victims seek help from their GPs.
- Four out of 10 victims seek medical help on at least five occasions.
- There are an estimated 3–4 million incidents of domestic violence in London alone every year.
- Violence increases in severity and frequency over time to about two attacks per week per woman.
- In one study, violence to female partners was found to comprise 25 per cent of recorded assaults.
- Victims suffer for an average of seven years before being able to leave for good.

Many women stay in a violent relationship, or return to it, simply to provide a roof over their children's heads, and to try to conform to society's expectations of a 'happy family'. Still others stay out of fear of reprisal on themselves or their children, and because they simply have nowhere else to go. Most women have lost their friends out of embarrassment, and through their partners' powerfully enforced desire to curtail their social lives, a behaviour that almost always accompanies violence. It has also been argued that such women suffer from post-traumatic stress syndrome, or are so brainwashed by the frequent physical and emotional abuse that they can barely think for themselves let alone make the elaborate plans required to leave.

Violence in families can also be directed at children, with tragic cases of such abuse brought regularly to public attention. Something in the order of 30 children in every 10 000 are recorded as 'at risk', with 32 500 listed in this way in 1993. In 1990 Childline counselled some 8600 victims of sexual abuse.

Case history 2.2

Beth, who is aged 42, looked thin and gaunt as she hobbled into surgery with a badly sprained ankle, which she explained was sustained at self-defence classes. Diagnosis and treatment were straightforward enough until, in the course of the consultation, she was asked why she was learning self-defence. She burst into tears and took some encouragement to explain that her husband was about to be released from jail after a three-year sentence for assaulting her. She had been abused by him throughout their entire married life, but had finally had enough and reported him to the police after his last vicious beating. Now she cannot sleep, cannot eat, and smokes far too much. She has moved house, but he has threatened to find her and come after her and her daughter as soon as he is released.

Social conditions

All doctors know how stressful people find problem neighbours, unemployment, noise, debt or overcrowding. These situations can happen at any time to anyone from any social background.

According to MIND, stressful life events are actually more common in socially or economically deprived groups. Indeed, people who are disadvantaged are even more likely to suffer from stress, just as they are from all mental health problems. It is easy to see how this may be so. In addition to all the problems just mentioned, they experience raised incidences of poverty, infant mortality, physical morbidity and mortality.

> Resolve not to be poor: whatever you have, spend less. Poverty is a great enemy to human happiness; it destroys liberty . . .
>
> (Samuel Johnson 1709–1784)

In areas officially designated as 'deprived', admission rates to psychiatric hospitals are three times above the national average. In a 1978 study, Brown and Harris found that 83 per cent of a group of women who were depressed had had previous traumatic life events or major continuing difficulties prior to the onset of the condition.

As if all of this distress is not enough, urban areas are associated with a higher incidence of social problems, such as youth and adult crime and families with difficulties. It has been estimated that 22 per cent of preschool children in urban areas will have behavioural problems. There is a higher incidence of behavioural disturbance in urban schoolchildren and adolescents.

Case history 2.3

Karen lives in an inner-city deprived area. She is aged just 21 and lives with the father of her 6-year-old son and 2-year-old daughter. She comes in to the surgery quietly and sits down with a sigh. Her mother is looking after her daughter so that she can ask the doctor for help with her nerves. Karen is constantly exhausted and on edge, and snaps at the children. She is scared that one day she will hit them too hard. The 2-year-old child has frequent tantrums, which seem to be getting worse, and the 6-year-old is bedwetting every night. Her boyfriend has been unemployed since she met him; he leaves everything to her and goes out to the pub every night. She asks if the GP can give her something to calm her down.

Housing

Shelter takes the view that anyone who does not have decent, secure and affordable housing is homeless. Based on this defintion, in England in 1994 over 127 000 households were homeless, with 8600 people estimated to be sleeping rough.

This does not include the 420 000 households whose mortgages were in arrears in 1994 and were at risk of becoming homeless; 49 000 homes were repossessed in the same year. The 1990s have also seen the new phenomenon of negative equity, whereby the mortgage that people are paying off is higher than the value of the house.

Case history 2.4

Raj, his wife and two small children are living in bed-and-breakfast accommodation, as he lost his job with the local council and the building society repossessed their house. Raj consults his doctor complaining of anxiety and chest pain. The whole family lives in an 8 by 12-foot room with no cooking facilities and a bathroom shared with 10 others. After breakfast, they have to stay away from the hotel until five o'clock in the evening. They have to carry all their belongings around with them because one of the other residents has been thieving from the rooms.

Crime

Crime and the fear of crime are constantly on people's minds. The majority of women will not walk alone in the streets after dark, and, if driving alone, are scared to accept offers of help from a passing 'good samaritan' if their car breaks down. Parents accompany their children everywhere. We even hesitate before approaching a lost or crying child in the street in case we are accused of molesting or attempting to abduct the child. People park their cars uncertain whether they will be intact or even still there on their return. Elderly people are constantly on edge at every noise, and wary of every group of young boys they pass in the street. The expression 'daylight robbery' has taken on a frightening ring of truth. This is a picture of danger on every corner and threat at every turn: the very stuff of stress.

Some of these fears are in fact unfounded, but that does not stop people having them. No matter how unlikely it is to happen to us, press and media coverage still beam heinous acts of crime in glorious technicolour and vivid detail into our homes on the hour every hour. For this and other reasons the old 'it will never happen to me' adage has been replaced for many by the certainty of 'if it can happen to them, it can happen to me'.

Although our fears may be exaggerated in some cases by media hype, the common perception of a rising problem is unnervingly borne out by official statistics. People do not even need to see these statistics to know this, because crime, particularly burglary and theft, is happening to them and their families, neighbours and friends on a regular basis.

In the 1990s, one in five of us is a victim of crime every year in the UK. According to government statistics, recorded crimes have risen from 1.6 million in 1970 to 5.4 million in 1993. The 1994 British Crime Survey of 10 000 households also takes unrecorded crime into account and suggests that 18 million crimes against individuals and their properties were committed in 1993. The vast majority of these crimes involve burglary and car and other theft, with only 5 per cent involving violent and sexual offences. Most of this crime is carried out by young men.

This is therefore not an imagined but a real fear, especially for those who live alone. It is a constant source of fearful anticipation, and, for one in five people every year, the fear becomes a reality with all the stress and emotional suffering of actually being a victim. Life for the victims may never be quite the same again.

Case history 2.5

Jacob is aged 58 and has recently been widowed, after nursing his wife for six months. He has just moved to a ground-floor flat allocated to him by the council, as this is all he can afford. He is on invalidity benefit for a heart condition; his wife's job had been his main source of income. He hardly hears from his two sons these days, as they had a disagreement years ago; he finds it very lonely. The other night, after he had gone to bed, he heard someone trying to open the kitchen window. He phoned the police, but they did not find anyone. That was three months ago, and he is still unable to sleep because of listening for noises. When he does fall asleep, he wakes up in a panic and can hardly catch his breath.

Suicide

We should never be in any doubt that stress is a most serious problem with potentially fatal consequences. Every two hours someone commits suicide in the UK, and, according to MIND and the World Health

Organization, social problems producing family stress are crucial factors in suicide risk. In most European countries, suicide comes within the 10 most common causes of death.

Unemployment has been found to be a leading factor, especially among young adults. For those in employment, farmers, pharmacists and veterinary surgeons are most at risk of suicide, partly because of access to the means of carrying out the act.

According to the Samaritans, the sharpest rise in suicide is amongst young men aged from 15 to 24 years, who are now seven times more likely to commit suicide than their female counterparts. Suicide is the second most common cause of death for young men. In 1995, this was attributed by Carol Lee, writing in *The Herald,* to a well of unspoken anger brought about by a lack of identity and financial insecurity.

An ageing population

Whatever decade of life a person has just completed, it can cause trauma and stress as he or she comes to terms with a changing identity. Even reaching the age of 30 or 40 years can have these effects. Mid-life can also be particularly difficult for both men and women, when they have to come to terms with having stopped growing up, and having begun to grow old, perhaps with ambitions not yet achieved and the meaning of life not yet worked out.

Youth is a malady of which one becomes cured a little every day.
(Benito Mussolini, on his 50th birthday)

When old age is reached, new problems can arise, many of which incur stress both for the elderly people themselves and for others in a society where there is little respect for older people. All doctors know that the proportion of elderly people is increasing. Even as younger people approach retirement, they are worrying about what will happen if they need care, as this burden may well fall on their children. Over 6 per cent of people aged over 65, and as many as 25 per cent of those aged over 80 suffer from dementia. When such care is required, stressful conflict among siblings and between the generations is often the outcome. In 1990, 3.7 million adults were caring for another person; most of these carers were women. Only 4 per cent of those who were over 65 years were in institutional care.

This is not the only problem. Within Europe as a whole, the number of elderly people living alone is increasing, with the attendant fear of crime, financial hardship, boredom, emptiness and social isolation that this can involve, and which is, again, the very stuff of stress. In 1991, 60 per cent of those aged over 80 years in the UK lived alone. An added twist to this is that, with increasing rates of divorce and remarriage, families are becoming increasingly fragmented and important social contact with grandchildren can be lost. As today's children grow up, they may even find that they have four or more sets of grandparents who are in need of care.

The days of the intact extended family, with the respected figure of the grandmother or grandfather sitting in their permanent place beside the fire, are over, and with them have gone freedom from worry and social support for many older people.

Carers

According to MIND, in 1995 there were 6 million carers in Britain. That means that one adult in seven was looking after someone who was ill, frail or disabled. Only 4 per cent of those aged over 65 were in institutional care. Most of these carers are women, and they are often discriminated against in terms of services:

> A study of 172 carers showed that 75 per cent of sons and 68 per cent of husbands received home help support as compared with only 4 per cent of mothers, 20 per cent of wives and 24 per cent of daughters. (MIND, 1995)

Doctors are only too aware of the unbearable and prolonged stress that can be placed on such carers. Sadly, one outcome of this can by physical abuse. Relate estimates that up to half a million old people may be at risk of physical abuse every year.

Racism

According to the 1991 Census, 5.5 per cent of the UK population belong to ethnic minorities. This is a significant minority, who are often the target of racist behaviour, some of it violent and extremely unpleasant. This is obviously a source of persistent, pervasive and long-term stress for those affected. It will also bite particularly hard because of the lack of control that the victims often feel they have over it. Some ethnic minorities, particularly those of Afro-Caribbean and Asian origin, are also more likely to be unemployed, or in lower paid work than their white counterparts. Black people are also over-represented in the homeless statistics. This means that the additional stress associated with poverty and deprivation already discussed is also likely to be added to the stress deriving from racism.

Alcohol

An information pack produced by Alcohol Concern (1993) states, 'As a nation, we spend more on alcoholic drinks than clothes, hospitals or schools: almost £16 billion a year.'

Alcohol use is both a cause and an outcome of stress. The use and abuse of alcohol leaves behind it a trail of untold suffering and stress. Here is some information provided by Alcohol Concern:

- The total cost to the UK in 1990 was £2461 million.
- The cost to general practice in 1990 was £2.8 million.
- It is estimated that, in 1993, 550 people died due to drinking and driving; 14 500 were casualties.
- Over 5200 pints of beer are consumed every minute.
- Ten people commit a drink-related crime of violence every hour.
- Every hour, 243 people are admitted to hospitals with alcohol-related problems.
- Every hour, three people die from drink-related causes.

Stress can also come from 'good' events

It would be wrong to leave the topic of life stress without addressing the fact that it is not only the negative events of life that can cause stress. Even events that are welcome can do so. This is because even happy events, such as a wedding, a new house or a promotion, involve a number of factors such as change, a feeling of lack of control, or time pressure, which can all cause stress. Who would not worry about the threat of being homeless if a new house cannot be found before having to leave the present one? Arranging a wedding or a holiday involves time pressure to make sure it all will be all right on the day, and worrying about what might unexpectedly go wrong. Most positive life events involve change, which we have noted to be stressful.

Workplace stress

Far and away the best prize that life offers is the chance to work hard at work worth doing.

(Theodore Roosevelt, 1903)

The third factor in the stress equation is workplace stress. This is coming more and more to the forefront in general practice, not least among GPs themselves. Emphasis on job satisfaction, as referred to so aptly by Roosevelt in 1903, has now given way to long hours, short-term contracts, new methods of working, and constant change, which, taken together, have brought about a sea change in working life in the UK today. The unemployed are stressed because they do not have a job, and the workforce is stressed because they do. What is the answer?

There is of course no easy answer, and no magic wand that will make workplace stress just disappear. As with life stresses, it is largely an outcome of the nature of the UK today, and doctors can do little about that, except deal with its casualties. The main responsibility surely lies with the employer. Specific skills for both employers and employees to use to manage workplace stress will be suggested in Chapter 4.

High and low stress occupations

Professor Cary Cooper and his colleagues have carried out a wide-ranging study of over 100 occupations, and ranked them according to their level of stress. A selection of their findings is as follows:

- Above average stress
  - Pilot;
  - Doctor;
  - Police officer;
  - Journalist;
  - Prison officer;
  - Nurse/midwife;
  - Social worker;
  - Teacher;
  - Psychologist;
  - Miner;
  - Manager;
  - Construction worker;
  - Dentist.
- Below average stress
  - Photographer;
  - Librarian;
  - Biochemist;
  - Laboratory technician;
  - Hairdresser;
  - Radiographer;
  - Engineer;
  - Dietician;
  - Insurance worker;
  - Speech therapist;
  - Optician.

Square pegs in round holes

Having just listed high and low stress jobs, this requires some further qualification. It is not quite so simple as that. No matter what the job is, if it does not match your personality, you will feel stressed by it. The outgoing person, who thrives on new activities and meeting new people, would probably find it hard to cope with work as a laboratory technician or a truck driver. The shrinking violet would probably find life impossible as a double-glazing salesperson or an actor. We will see other examples of this in Chapter 3 (Case histories 3.4 and 3.7), where new requirements such as team-working or speaking up in groups is a potential area of difficulty for many people.

The dilemma today is that, with a high rate of unemployment, people are often obliged to take whatever job they can find, whether it suits their personality or not. Jobs are no longer static in the way that they used to be. Jobs change, sometimes rapidly, and often out of all recognition. Employers want a flexible workforce, and there is no such thing as a job for life. With the threat of unemployment, people have to accept changes to their jobs that do not match their personalities. The outcome is often stress.

Causes of workplace stress

Other causes of stress at work are many and varied. The most commonly cited include deadlines, poor internal communications and excessive hours. A check list of possible sources follows; doctors will probably find much to identify with here:

- Conditions of the job
  - Uncertainty and insecurity;
  - Poor status, low pay, no promotion prospects;
  - Long or unsociable hours;
  - Shift work, upsetting circadian rhythm;
  - Insufficient back-up;
  - Unnecessary procedures;
  - Travel to and from work (cramped unpunctual trains, long journeys, city driving, etc.);
  - Working from home;
  - Taking work home;
  - Overwork or underwork;
  - Time pressure, especially if prolonged;
  - Lack of variety;
  - Demands made on private and social life;
  - Doing job below level of competence;
  - Attending meetings;
  - Amount of travelling;
  - Ease of contact – e-mail, fax, bleepers, car-phones, mobile phones – even at home.

- Your employer
  - Organizational problems;
  - Your beliefs conflicting with your employer's;
  - Staff shortages.

- The job itself
  - Unclear role;
  - Role conflict;
  - Powerlessness or feeling trapped;
  - Unrealistic deadlines;
  - Inability to get a job finished;
  - Difficult clients or patients;
  - Incompetent colleagues;
  - Insufficient training;
  - Emotional involvement with clients;
  - The responsibilities;
  - Inability to help or to act effectively;
  - Keeping up with new developments or new technology;
  - Having to move home often.

- The job environment
  - Noisy or cramped conditions;
  - Excessive heat or humidity;
  - Presence of toxic or dangerous materials.

- Your superiors
  - Clashing with superiors;
  - Inadequate leadership.

- Your subordinates
  - Inadequate training;
  - Clashes or difficulties with them;
  - Having to discipline them.

- Communication with others
  - Isolation;
  - Poor communication or none;
  - Conflict with colleagues;
  - Unnecessary battles.

- Your personality and expectations
  - Perfectionist;
  - Low tolerance for stress;
  - Intolerant of certain behaviours in others (e.g. tidiness, punctuality);
  - Type A personality (see Chapter 3);
  - Lack of confidence;
  - Not assertive: either too passive, or too aggressive.

- Problems particularly affecting women
  - Dual role of career and home or family;
  - First woman in the job;
  - Having to travel or stay in hotels alone;
  - Being conspicuously different;
  - Sexism and sexual harassment;
  - Male colleagues can feel threatened;
  - Promotion can be difficult.

Outcomes of workplace stress for the employer

Stress at work is not just a problem for the employee. It has costly repercussions for the employer too, with an annual cost to UK industry of £4100 million. Here are some of the factors contributing to that cost:

- Absenteeism due to stress, and other illnesses caused by stress;
- Absenteeism due to alcohol or drugs;
- High staff turnover;
- Poor time-keeping;
- Underperformance of workforce;
- Poor relationships between workers or with customers;
- Increased accident rate;
- Litigation for stress-related illness.

Summary

- People are, in general, more stressed today, for a number of reasons.
- An individual's total stress is a combination of life stress and workplace stress.
- The sum of these is probably greater than the two separately.
- Some people are more vulnerable to stress than others through no fault of their own.
- Workplace stress arises from many different causes.

3

Individual vulnerability to stress

Many patients will present in the surgery with difficulties related to the life and workplace stresses that have been discussed in the previous chapter. In one morning, a GP may see the long-term unemployed middle-aged man who has irritable bowel syndrome, the single mother of three small children from a deprived area, who is underweight and has frequent tension headaches, and the young overworked executive who is unable to sleep. It is easy to envisage and understand why these patients are having problems, but we also know that there are many others who cope with similar situations without experiencing stress. In that same morning, the GP may also see other patients who are experiencing stress from a situation that the doctor finds hard to see as stressful. What is the difference? Are some people more vulnerable to stress than others? Are they weaker people?

The simple answer is that, yes, some people are more vulnerable to stress in certain circumstances, but no, they are certainly not weak people.

We have already seen that, for some people, autonomic arousal does occur much more easily due to their constitutional make-up. They clearly have no control over this, and can no more be blamed for it than for having blue or green eyes, or a genetic disposition towards diabetes or heart disease. These people would have been the survivors in prehistoric times, when physical threat was frequent, and may even have been admired greatly for their lightning reaction to danger. From experience of hearing the descriptions of the day-to-day lives of many such patients, the only possible conclusion to reach is that these are in fact very brave people. Their bodies are frequently on the alert, mobilized for action that is never needed, producing very unpleasant symptoms including hyperventilation, tension and anxiety. They can do little about this, but most manage to struggle on courageously, living their lives and trying to maintain some degree of normality. If we can for a moment think of a situation that makes us even mildly anxious or fearful, then imagine such a feeling repeated frequently or constantly over weeks or months, and we may have some inkling of their experience. It may also be easier to understand their frequent visits to the surgery, and their urgent need of treatment.

In addition to constitutional variations, there are also wide individual differences in personality, coping style, social support and previous experience. Again, people also have little or no choice or control over these, but such factors can increase or reduce their vulnerability to stress in certain circumstances.

However, there is no definitive, across the board set of personal characteristics that is more or less likely to encourage stress, neither is there any intrinsic weakness or strength attached to them. It could be said that, in any particular culture, a different group of characteristics will increase vulnerability to stress. It really all depends on the particular mix of persons and situations. For some, it really could be considered to be a case of being the wrong person in the wrong place at the wrong time.

In many aspects of life today the personality characteristics of a perfectionist have a high propensity to induce stress. The perfectionist working in a job such as social work or teaching, which often requires the prioritizing and limiting of the amount of work able to be tackled due to restraints of time and resources, may find themselves stressed because they cannot deal with everything perfectly. On the other hand, all things being equal, the perfectionist working as a pharmacist or a radiologist, where performance must be as complete and mistake-free as possible, is much more likely to be stress free.

It is much the same for coping strategies. The person who uses denial to deal with a debt problem will simply find that the problem gets worse and more stressful, but, if the same person's wife dies suddenly, then denying the reality of the death immediately after the event may have a protective effect from a stress reaction that might otherwise have been overwhelming.

There is also now evidence to suggest that being part of a social network provides a protection against stressful life events, and against stress-related ill health. This social support can come from family, friends, work colleagues or the local community. The more extensive the support, the better. Those with little support of this kind are vulnerable to stress, and find difficulty in coping with the daily hassles and problems of life.

No one is immune to stress. No matter what our constitutional make-up, personality characteristics, coping style, social support or previous experience, there will still be situations that can bring about stress. Even Baroness Thatcher, the 'Iron Lady', who appeared to cope with everything that being Prime Minister could demand of her, was visibly stressed in that famous television footage of her leaving Number 10 Downing Street so suddenly and unexpectedly in November 1990, when she was replaced by John Major.

Professor Cary Cooper's 'stress equation' was introduced in Chapter 2:

$$\text{Life stress} + \text{Work stress} + \text{Individual vulnerability} = \text{Stress symptoms/outcomes}$$

Life stress and workplace stress have already been discussed, so we now turn to look in more detail at those factors other than constitution that contribute to individual vulnerability: personality, previous experience and coping style. Doctors treating stress do not need to have knowledge of all the details presented here, but a general grasp of the overall picture will make approaching the patient and coming to a diagnosis that much easier. The information given here may also be useful for doctors to assess their own personal vulnerability to stress.

Personality

Tempora mutantur, et nos mutamur in illis (times change, and we change with them).

(Emperor Lothar I, 795–855)

Even today, the argument still continues about whether personality is a constant, stable entity, or whether it can change. People can exhibit different aspects of their personalities in different situations: doting father one minute; authoritarian manager the next; indulgent lover the next. Do people not change over time: angry and moody at 18; full of initiative, drive and urgency at 42; cautious, methodical and concerned about the environment at 65? Arguments can be made both for this kind of changing personality with the situation and over time, and also for more permanence in our general disposition. If too much time is spent on the vagaries of this ongoing argument, there will be no opportunity to explain the undoubted link between certain personality character-istics and stress. In order to simplify matters, let us assume for the moment that, in a given situation at some point in time, an individual behaves and thinks in accordance with certain fairly constant person-ality traits, and that this will affect their experience of stress.

Type A and Type B personalities

Probably the most well-known model linking personality and stress was developed by two cardiologists, Meyer Friedman and Ray Rosenman in 1974. They described two extremes of personality and thinking style described as Type A and Type B. Type A individuals are prone to stress and it is suggested that, over time, this type of behaviour can lead to premature coronary artery disease. Those with a Type B personality are less stress prone, and therefore less likely to succumb to stress-related illness. Two examples of behaviour and thinking follow.

Case history 3.1

Jenny is aged 32, and manager of a small but growing electronics firm. She jumps out of bed in the morning as soon as the alarm goes off, eats toast and drinks strong black coffee at the same time as reading some papers from work, before grabbing her brief case and the other paperwork she was working on last night and dashing off to the car. It does not start first time, so she mutters angrily about how she never has time to arrange its service. She has barely allowed time to get to work in time before the first of numerous important meetings, which, if it goes well, could mean the clinching of a very important deal. Mercifully, the car then purrs into life, and she heaves a sigh of relief and sets off. Within minutes she comes to roadworks and slowly moving traffic, and another car pulls in sharply in front of her. 'Stupid fool', she barks, banging on the horn. Her anger rises and so does her heart rate. She sighs again. Where has this traffic come from so unexpectedly? Why did she not leave earlier? Tension persists and increases throughout her body, she grips the wheel tightly and turns up the volume of the music on the radio. She reaches work late, and bellows at her secretary to get her a coffee, and wants to know why she had not warned her about the roadworks.

Case history 3.2

John is aged 37 and manages a small but growing knitwear factory. He wakes to the sound of relaxing music on his radio, and gets up slowly and stretches. There is an important meeting today, so he has allowed extra time to get to work in case of traffic. After sitting down to breakfast and a chat with his wife, he glances through the business pages of the paper then walks out to the car, noticing that the roses need pruning as he passes them. The car has just had its regular service and bursts into life at the first turn of the key. Soon he is driving in single line traffic; he starts when the car alongside him suddenly pulls in front of him. He decides that the driver must be in a hurry to get somewhere, then forgets about it. On arriving at work, he has time to look over the day's appointments before his secretary arrives.

These are, of course, rather stereotypical views of the two extremes, Jenny being a Type A and John a Type B, but the different styles of thinking and behaving clearly have repercussions. Scenes such as these will be re-enacted in countless homes, offices, schools and doctors' practices every day.

The belief system and behaviour of those with a Type A personality increases their vulnerability to stress. They find it hard to relax without feeling guilty; their self-worth is bound up with their achievements, and they are therefore personally pledged to success and accomplishment in everything they do. Anything delaying these goals therefore incurs frustration and anger. There are no allowances made for mistakes, or for flexibility. This produces frequent arousal due to a hectic pace and a persistent appraisal of threat, which is untempered by breaks for relaxation of any kind.

Most individuals will actually exhibit a mixture of Type A and Type B behaviours. The following behaviours are typical of Type A and can help to identify its elements in patients and in doctors:

- Doing everything quickly: talking, eating, walking;
- Impatience, especially in queues;
- Strongly competitive;
- Not planning time realistically (self-imposed deadlines that are too tight);
- Emphasizing key words in normal speech;
- Being unable to relax or do nothing without a sense of guilt;
- Hurrying other people's speech by finishing their sentences for them;
- Frequently doing two or more things at once;
- Working towards poorly defined goals;
- Becoming oblivious to beauty and things of interest around them;
- Material success is very important;
- A chronic sense of time urgency, and arranging more and more into less and less time;
- Hostility and aggression, especially to others of Type A;
- Using gestures such as a clenched fist or banging on the table for emphasis.

Friedman and Rosenman (1974) describe the following character-istics, which are typical of Type B behaviours:

- Being free of Type A characteristics;
- Feeling no need to impress others with their achievements;
- Able to relax without feeling guilty;
- No sense of time urgency;
- No in-built hostility or competitiveness;
- Slow, calm and attentive;
- Warm, medium volume voice.

Since most people display a combination of Type A and Type B behaviours and thinking style, it is useful to be aware of how these might contribute to the overall picture of a patient's experience of stress.

The obsessional personality

Here we are not talking about the person who exhibits pathological behaviour such as obsessional hand-washing or cleaning. Many people have an element of obsessional behaviour within their personalities, which is entirely nonpathological. The perfectionist mentioned earlier is an example of this, being someone who cannot tolerate mistakes in themselves or even in others. Other obsessional individuals might set standards for themselves and others in terms of punctuality, conscientiousness or conformity. Obsessionality is characterized by an inability to tolerate variations from their chosen way of doing things, or a chosen subject for sole consideration. Such individuals have very fixed thinking, and are strongly resistant to change and new ideas. They are most at home in a situation where everything is precise and predictable, so, if their environment does not complement this obsessionality, stress will be the outcome.

Case history 3.3

Frances is an office worker who keeps everything neat and tidy and in its place at all times, and cannot tolerate the slightest untidiness. All is well, until a new office junior, Brian, starts work, who refuses to comply. He says he works better with a muddle around him. Frances now finds she is losing weight because she has lost her appetite, and her old migraine problem has recurred. She visits her GP complaining of stress at work.

Case history 3.4

Joseph is the 50-year-old manager of a factory, and is used to an authoritarian system, which has always allowed him to determine and put into place his own choice of production methods. Team working has just been introduced into the company and the production methods are now to be decided upon by a team of which he is only one member. He finds it difficult to accept the views of others on how things should be done. He now feels tired all the time and has begun to wake up with anxiety attacks during the nights prior to team meetings. He visits his GP complaining of stress at work.

These two patients are both complaining of workplace stress; each has a very different problem, but both having an origin within themselves, rather than in the workplace.

The 'hardy' personality

In 1979, Suzanne Kobasa developed her theory of 'hardiness' with respect to the ability of an individual to withstand stress. After studying a group of executives who were experiencing similar high levels of stress, she found that certain personality characteristics made it less likely that the stress would result in mental or physical ill health. She asserted that this group of attributes comprised what she defined as 'hardy' personality. These attributes, 'the three Cs' are:

- *Commitment*: an active involvement in and a commitment to a range of areas of life, such as work, family, friends and institutions;
- *Control*: a feeling of being in control of one's life, and able to influence events;
- *Challenge*: an acceptance of change as inevitable, and being open and willing to try new things that are embraced as a challenge.

Those who have a sense of commitment, a feeling of control and enjoy change and new activities are therefore less likely to experience stress. In contrast to this, those who have little personal commitment, feel a lack of control over their lives, and enjoy stability rather than change are vulnerable to stress. It is probably fair to add that this scenario is specific to a life in which change is endemic; in a society in which there is constant unpredictable change, such as in western society, the three Cs will provide stressproofing. If times change and life becomes very predictable and unchanging, the whole situation might be very different.

The personality with a sense of control

Kobasa includes a sense of control in her hardy personality, and the whole idea of control seems to be a vital one in any discussion about stress. It seems intuitively correct that, faced with a threatening or difficult situation over which we have no control, stress is likely to be that much greater than if we feel able to do something about it. But sometimes awareness of whether or not we have control is less clear-cut than we might think.

Case history 3.5

Kevin has just begun a course in biochemistry at a large university and is finding it increasingly difficult to cope with the work. The lectures are complicated and the pace is faster than he had expected. It is difficult to get to know people, as the lectures are attended by so many students. He now feels, after only six weeks, that the work is totally out of his control and that he just is not up to it. He has also been feeling panicky and light-headed during lectures, and has had to leave for some fresh air on several occasions. He is sure that he will have to give up at Christmas and is angry that life is not fair. Why do these things always happen to him?

Case history 3.6

Liz is on the same course as Kevin, and has noticed him having to go out during lectures. She found the sudden increase in pace and level a shock at first, but decided she would need to put in more study to keep up, and that seemed to work. She also made a point of talking to other students, and discovered that they all felt the same. She finds the library staff helpful in finding books on the parts of the course that are difficult to understand, and the tutorials are very useful for asking questions. She is confident that she can cope with the course and is enjoying the experience.

As early as 1966, J. B. Rotter was describing the significance of people's perceptions of whether or not they have control over situations. He introduced the concept of the locus of control and would have described Kevin as having an external locus of control, and Liz as having an internal locus of control. That is Liz feels she has her own, internal control over what happens to her, and that her actions and decisions have an effect on her life experience. So she works harder, finds out how others are feeling, and gets further help from the library. Kevin, on the other hand, feels that he has little influence or control over events, and that external factors such as fate or chance are largely responsible for what happens to him, so he sits back and takes whatever happens to him as if he has no power to alter it. Kevin is therefore likely to experience stress and appear in the doctor's surgery for help, whilst Liz is not.

Rotter's view was that those with an external locus of control are more vulnerable to stress in most situations, and that such individuals tend to hold some or all of the following beliefs:

- Luck and chance play a crucial role in life.
- Success is determined by being in the right place at the right time.
- What happens to us is predestined.
- In our lives, we are all subject to forces that we cannot control.

Once again, it is worth pointing out that the issue of control may be one that arises from life in a culture in which much of our daily life is unpredictable and outwith our control.

Previous experience

> Our deeds still travel with us from afar,
> And what we have been, makes us what we are.
>
> (George Eliot, 1819–1880)

There are many and varied views about how previous experience affects the way people react in particular situations. However, it does seem fair to assume that people learn from experience and that this learning can affect their future behaviour. Let's consider some examples.

Confidence

Case history 3.7

Gita never got on with her father, who was a very strict and aggressive man, who held very fixed views. For as long as she could remember, whenever she expressed a view of her own, he aggressively and unkindly criticized it and tore it to shreds. She grew up lacking in confidence about herself, especially about saying what she thought to others. She was intelligent and able, and easily obtained a degree in business administration, but when she started her first job in management for a major retailer, she found herself feeling under stress and mildly depressed. The job often required her to express her opinion in meetings and to colleagues. She found herself sweating and trembling at these times, and she would often stammer and forget what she was saying when asked for her views or advice.

Gita's previous experience meant that she perceived herself to be less able than she was and to fear criticism. She therefore found situations in which she had to express an opinion to others to be very stressful. Feeling stressed when speaking up at meetings or making presentations to colleagues is very commonly due to lack of confidence. This is often the result of family or educational experiences that have produced low self-esteem. This can, of course, also reach pathological proportions, when acute anxiety or even a phobic response may be produced in such situations. In terms of stress, recent changes in working conditions and methods have often meant that people who are unaccustomed to do so are having to speak up in this way or to work in teams. This often means that a job that was previously no problem for an individual can easily become stressful.

Other attitudes

Confidence in oneself is only one example of a range of factors that can be influenced by previous experience, all of which have repercussions in making people vulnerable to stress. For example, people may become particularly suspicious of others, pessimistic, prone to feelings of guilt, withdrawn, dependent on others, or even hostile and aggressive. In the wrong place or at the wrong time, all of these behaviours can produce stress.

Previous experience of stress or negative life events

An individual who has experienced a number of negative life events is much more likely to suffer stress again for two reasons. David Barlow (1988) suggests that previous experience of uncontrollable and/or unpredictable life events can result in chronic anxious apprehension, even in the absence of a new stress, due to chronic overarousal. This is often the outcome of intermittent stress, especially of an uncontrollable nature. Secondly, any new stress is much more likely to trigger an exaggerated stress response, as the individual's autonomic system has now become sensitized to stress.

Strategies acquired for coping with stress

Probably one of the most important things in people's previous experience is the coping strategies that they have learned to use when stressed. Knowing how to deal effectively with stress does not come naturally. It is during childhood and throughout life, when we have to deal with stress, that we develop strategies for coping with it.

We acquire these strategies in the main by copying others, or by applying what we think is common sense, or using what we find works. If our parents reacted to stress by running about wringing their hands, or by bottling it all up, we may well do the same. After all, we learn how to tie our laces and to speak by copying the adults around us, so it is not surprising that we learn how to deal with stress in a similar way. We also learn ways of coping with stress from wider society. If people in general say that taking your mind off things is a useful thing to do, we are likely to give it a try, and, if it works, this will become part of our repertoire for dealing with stress.

Having said all this, sometimes a strategy may not really be a conscious choice at all. Many people automatically speed up or keep busy in response to stress, probably due to the autonomic changes that are initiated, mobilizing the body for physical action. Other strategies, such as denial or projecting our feelings on to others, may be equally unconscious; these are likely to be largely the outcome of our psychological make-up.

Some of these coping strategies are helpful, some are unhelpful. As we have seen, some, such as denial, are helpful in some situations and

unhelpful in others. Many patients appearing in the surgery are lik
be using coping strategies that are, at best, not helping and, at w ..,
may even be making matters worse. Learning stress management is
about learning a range of helpful strategies to deal with stress in
different situations. In later chapters we will look at these in detail and
see how the GP can make use of them. Meanwhile, it is useful to be
aware of the kinds of unhelpful strategies that patients might already be
using to cope with their stress when they arrive at the surgery looking
for the doctor's advice. Both the doctor and the patient require to
recognize and take stock of these before more effective strategies are
offered. Let us now take a closer look at these.

Unhelpful coping strategies

Increased substance use
Doctors are familiar with patients who drink or smoke to excess. This
is often an outcome of even a low level of stress in their lives. The use
of nonprescription drugs is also a common reaction to stress. Not only
is this behaviour counterproductive in terms of stress but the added risks
to health are also obvious.

Eating
Many people have learned in childhood to associate feeling relaxed and
at ease with eating. It is easy to see how that can happen when sweets
are used as rewards and to reduce the pain of a grazed knee. Comfort
eating is therefore a common feature of stress, with the attendant health
risks if weight and sugar intake begins to increase as a result.

Working longer, harder and faster
Many people are stressed because they have too much to do, both paid
and unpaid work, in too little time. An understandable and common
reaction to this is to work harder and work longer hours, in order to get
everything done, usually with fewer and shorter breaks. People skip
lunch, or have lunch-time meetings, work late, skip days off to catch up
with the work, take work home, miss out on holidays, and so on. To add
to the pressure, many realistically have no option as their jobs and
livelihood, or their family's well-being may depend on getting through
the workload. However, all of these coping strategies will actually make
matters worse. The body rapidly becomes tired, drained and open to
disease, and also becomes less resistant to stress. A vicious circle will
be initiated, whereby the individual will feel more stressed and probably
become physically and psychologically ill, and yet still nothing has
been done to tackle the original situation.

Overactivity
Another common reaction to stress is to keep very busy with other things, sometimes to excess. Every minute of the day can be filled with work, hobbies, clubs, sport or socializing. This can be an outcome of arousal, and a feeling that you simply have to keep going, or it can be a way of avoiding the stressful situation. All of this activity usually means that the problem itself is being avoided and not dealt with, and arousal is being maintained over longer and longer periods.

Denial
There are various forms of denial; most of them are harmful in most situations. The exception to this is the temporary denial which can exert a protective effect in the case of a serious trauma such as sexual abuse, rape or the death of a loved one. When in denial, an individual may:

• Bottle everything up inside;
• Pretend it is not a problem;
• Reason it all away;
• Hide his or her feelings;
• Carry on as if nothing had happened;
• Put on a brave face.

Denial is particularly common amongst those who see admitting a problem with stress as a sign of weakness. This is an outcome of a society that values coping and success and sees an inability to cope as failure. In any event, denial means the situation causing the stress itself is not being tackled; in the long term this can result in exhaustion, stress-related disease, anxiety and depression, or sudden outbursts of rage or grief. Many cases of anxiety or depression are the result of unresolved grief or trauma due to continuing denial, possibly for years. This is particulary common in adults who were sexually abused as children.

Escapism
Many people simply escape from their problematic situation, rather than dealing with it. They might move from job to job, and from relationship to relationship, never attempting to sort out the difficulties. This can place the person in something of a downward spiral, with no permanency in any aspect of life. Also, if a situation occurs from which there is no escape, such as a death, this individual will experience particularly acute stress.

Taking it out on other people
This takes the form of either blaming others for everything, or taking out on them the feelings of anger and frustration. Loved ones will often be the target for this type of anger. Apart from relieving some of these pent-up emotions, little benefit is gained by this, and much damage can be done to relationships.

Summary

Some patients will be more vulnerable to stress, through no fault of their own, but for the following reasons:

- A labile autonomic system;
- Lack of social support;
- Previous experience of stress or negative life events;
- Personality characteristics that are detrimental to their situation;
- Feeling that they have no control over their situation;
- A lack of a sense of challenge and commitment;
- A lack of confidence due to previous experiences;
- Using unhelpful coping strategies.

4

How to manage stress

The last two chapters have explained the extraordinary variation in the aetiology of stress. Our task now is to begin to think about how all this stress should be tackled. One of the most straightforward solutions would be to change society and the way we live today. However, this option remains closed to doctors, so we will have to make do with a range of stress management techniques instead, all of which can easily be made available to patients.

Knowing how to deal with stress does not come naturally to most people. As we have seen, patients will arrive at the surgery for all sorts of reasons. They will already be using coping strategies to deal with their stress; many of these tactics will be making matters worse. In fact, what we do automatically, or through common sense, can often be counterproductive. People might deny or try to escape from the problem, take it all out on someone else, or work too hard with no breaks. Unhelpful coping strategies of this kind have already been described in Chapter 3. Although these days most patients are well informed about the existence of stress, they are nevertheless floundering in a sea of misinformation and ignorance about how to deal with it. All they need from the GP is some clear, reliable and concrete advice.

Effective strategies for managing stress are set out in this chapter, along with more specific information about workplace stress. These strategies have developed mainly through practical use since the First World War, with a particular burgeoning of new techniques, probably from around the early 1970s. This was presumably the result of increasing stress throughout the western world. These techniques are described and explained in some detail here as background information for the GP. Later chapters will describe a range of health care professionals to whom patients may be referred for such advice, and also how the techniques might easily be adapted for straightforward use by the GP or other health care professional within primary care itself.

Doctors do not need to have a complete understanding of all of these techniques in order to make them available to their patients. The important thing to know is that these techniques are effective for many patients and that they can learn about them from a variety of sources.

A broad range of techniques is presented here, and this reflects the multifaceted nature of stress. However, an individual patient needs only to put into practice those techniques that are relevant to his or her particular situation, and which are found to be effective. Since Donald Meichenbaum put forward his plan for 'stress inoculation training' in 1974, most stress management advice has involved providing patients with information and explanation about stress, along with an armoury of techniques from which they can choose for themselves.

The GP will find that patients are surprisingly good at this. The patient with a chronic hyperventilation problem will find that the breathing exercises are hugely effective; the obsessive personality will think again about how they see the world and perhaps make changes that will reduce the stress; the excessive coffee drinker will buy decaffeinated coffee and feel much less hyperactive. Giving the patient control of his or her own strategies for managing stress not only eases the task of the GP but also increases the patient's sense of being in control of the situation. As we saw earlier, this can be a crucial factor in reducing stress. Having said that, many years of experience would suggest that the most powerful techniques for most patients involve a combination of relaxation, breathing exercises and gaining a better understanding about the causes and basic physiology of stress.

We now turn to a consideration of these and other techniques for managing stress. Though there is some overlap, they fall roughly into

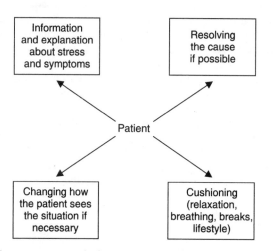

Figure 4.1 Stress management: the four processes involved.

the following categories, as shown in Figure 4.1:

- Providing information and explanation about stress;
- Resolving the cause of the stress;
- Cushioning the effects of stress;
- Changing how the person sees the situation.

The approach taken here is a retrospective one, in that we assume that stress is already being experienced by the patient. In a perfect world, everyone should learn about stress and how to manage it, so that they can do their best to avoid it and know what to do if it arises in themselves or in others.

Techniques used in the management of stress

Providing information and explanation

Allaying fears arising from ignorance and misinformation

> No passion so effectually robs the mind of all its powers of acting and reasoning as fear.
>
> (Edmund Burke, 1729–1797)

This aspect of managing stress is often underrated and may sometimes not even be included in stress management advice or courses. However, it can be a crucial component and is possibly even more relevant in primary care, where the GP has the knowledge and authority that the patient often needs to be convinced that the symptoms are not life-threatening and do have a straightforward explanation.

Magazines, television, radio and newspapers have all played their part in misinforming the public about stress and what can be done about it. Most either oversimplify or overcomplicate the subject. Television discussion programmes can leave the viewer feeling that there are a multiplicity of explanations about stress and that nobody really has any answers. Magazine articles can oversimplify and present the case from a biased point of view, suggesting that all will be well if the reader uses the particular therapy they are advocating.

It is from this maelstrom of misinformation that the patient arrives seeking the doctor's help. The authority of the GP can therefore be usefully harnessed to clarify and explain what stress is, and why the person is experiencing these particular symptoms. Patients will be more convinced and consoled by this than by any other source of information.

Armed with this new-found understanding, the patient should also be prevented from entering the vicious circle whereby more stress is built on top of the original stress through anxiety about the symptoms themselves. This applies particularly to the psychological and behavioural symptoms of stress, which make many patients feel that they are going mad, and to the physical symptoms, which they associate with a threat to life.

Understanding and dealing with panic attacks
Another symptom that benefits greatly from this approach is panic attacks. A panic attack is a very common outcome of stress. The fight or flight response is often triggered by events, or even by something as transient and unsubstantial as a fleeting thought, especially with a sensitized nervous system: 'What if I can't get this done in time?' or 'What if I can't pay those bills?'

Understanding what is happening, and what the patient can do about it, can defuse a situation which, if left untreated, can surprisingly quickly result in avoidance behaviour leading to life-restricting phobias such as agoraphobia, which is an increasingly common outcome of stress.

Case history 4.1

Kirsty walked into the consulting room, her face a mixture of fear and worry. She was aged 32, married and worked full-time. Her eyes were downcast and she trembled as she slowly and hesitantly explained that she was sure she was going mad. Yesterday at work she had 'come over all peculiar'. She could not think straight, was convinced something terrible was about to happen, and her heart had pounded. She had also had a feeling of acute panic, and had found herself rushing out of the office without explaining. The funny thing was that, as soon as she got home, she felt fine again. What was happening to her? Was this a nervous breakdown? What would everyone think? What if it should happen again? Gentle questioning revealed that she had been under pressure for some weeks as she was moving house, and had already bought a house, but could not sell her own. She was not sleeping well, and felt tired all the time.

Doctors will be aware of how frightening a panic attack like this can be for a patient. They feel the victim of a terrifying attack over which they appear to have absolutely no control. They are often convinced that they are going mad or are about to die. If the patient does not regain control over these attacks, which seem to them to strike out of the blue, the vicious circle will quickly, if not immediately, establish itself. Still higher levels of chronic arousal will be produced as they anticipate the next attack, and avoidance behaviour will be targeted on the situations that they fear may provoke an attack. The fleeting thought, 'What if I panic now?', can immediately instigate the feared attack. It becomes alarmingly easy then for a serious phobia to develop rapidly.

The approach to panic attacks is two-pronged. First, as described already, the level of stress is often substantially reduced simply by explaining the mechanism whereby patients feel the way they do. This is even more true for panic attacks. Once explained and understood, the fantasy of an unpredictable and terrifying attack can be transformed into the reality of a completely natural automatic defence mechanism. Secondly, patients must learn how they can deal with an attack as soon as they feel it coming on. This allows them to regain a feeling of having control over the situation, as well as being able to prevent a very distressing experience.

This can have a rapid and remarkable effect on a patient. One woman who was suffering from stress and panic attacks attended a seminar run by a local voluntary group. So unsteady was she that she required physical support to reach her seat to listen to an explanation of panic attacks being given by a clinical psychologist. She sat shaking at the back next to the door, hardly able to speak for anxiety. By the end of the explanation, she was in the front row confidently asking questions. The famous quotation from Franklin D. Roosevelt, 'We have nothing to fear but fear itself', comes easily to mind in this context.

Details on how patients can deal with panic are given in the text for a patient booklet in Appendix 5, but, generally speaking, patients must first have an explanation about the nature of panic attacks, and then learn two possible ways of dealing with them:

• Allowing the panic attack simply to blow itself out without reacting to it;
• Using relaxation or breathing exercises to reduce arousal as soon as they feel the panic attack coming on, thus severely curtailing its full effects, if not completely preventing the attack.

Most patients prefer the second method and find it very effective. A mnemonic of some kind, such as 'PAUSE', or 'CALM' is often used to help patients to remember what to do, given the sorts of disorientated thinking they may be experiencing at the time.

Resolving the cause of the stress

At its most basic, the simplest way to deal with stress quickly and effectively is to remove or eradicate its cause. If an individual finds his or her job or neighbourhood stressful and it is possible to move to another, then doing so will entirely remove the cause of the stress and the problem will be solved.

But, as doctors know, in most of the situations faced by their patients, removing the cause of stress is simple to say, but not so simple to do. People cannot just find another house or a new job, or find someone else to share the burden of a parent with dementia. As already mentioned in the discussion of coping strategies in the previous chapter, care must also be taken not to build up a pattern of avoidance behaviour in response to stressful situations, as this is unhelpful in the long term and can even encourage the development of a disabling and restrictive phobia. A severe stress reaction can also occur when the patient finds themselves faced with stress from which there is no escape.

However, many patients will already have explored these avenues before seeking help at the surgery. An abundance of support groups and advisory bodies is available today for people to consult for expert advice on their particular problem, and this can be greatly beneficial. Valuable expertise on such dilemmas as debt, failing relationships, housing, or legal matters is usually locally available, especially in areas of deprivation. Some patients do need encouragement to take the step of seeking such help, as many hold the view that this is an admission of an inability to cope on their own, which is a difficult admission to make in today's world. Simply coming to the doctor for help of this kind is itself something many find difficult to contemplate. This is particularly true of elderly people, many of whom feel that, since they came through a world war without succumbing to stress, they should be able to come through anything.

Unfortunately, as we have seen, it is often simply today's hectic everyday lifestyle, together with a lessening of family and community support, which is itself stressful. A whole range of regular hassles and difficulties add up to a great deal of stress, which is very difficult if not impossible to avoid or do something about. People therefore feel trapped and powerless, with little support or control over their lives, and this only adds to the stress they experience.

We have also seen that sometimes the cause of the stress lies within people themselves. They may have personality and other characteristics that increase their vulnerability to stress. Just as finding jobs for people and relieving poverty and deprivation is difficult to do, so changing such characteristics in order to remove stress can be a complicated and difficult task. If the individual has a labile autonomic nervous system, nothing can be done to change that, and cushioning from its effects is the best solution. Similarly if the individual's personality or thinking style, or that person's past history lays him or her open to stress, it can be difficult to alter this substantially without referral for more complex therapy. However, much can still be done to tackle these problems, even within the bounds of stress management, and this is covered in the section dealing with changing how people see the situation.

Becoming more assertive

Stressful situations often arise from people not being able to communicate their needs and wishes to others, both at work and in relationships. Like many other stress management techniques, assertiveness training developed largely in the 1970s and, although it has relevance in a much wider arena, it also has clear significance here. By making their behaviour more assertive, patients may be able to change a stressful situation into one that can be managed, and prevent other stressful situations from arising. Doctors may see this as a somewhat trendy idea, but assertiveness strikes at the very heart of most human relationships and dilemmas, and its effects on an individual can be profound and long-lasting. It can be particularly effective in relationship problems and in the workplace.

Here are some examples of people who are not being assertive, and who are likely to encourage stress for themselves; people who:

- Find they cannot say 'no' and become overburdened;
- Cannot speak up about their own needs to others;
- Are overbearing or aggressive to others;
- Get their own way by making others feel guilty;
- Cannot give criticism without devaluing the other person;
- Have to win at all costs.

Many stressful situations arise out of this type of poor interpersonal communication, whether at work, at home or elsewhere. This can affect all relationships from the most intimate to the most public. Improving assertiveness skills can therefore change a situation causing stress into one that is more manageable.

Assertiveness training is based on the premise that everyone is equal and has the same rights, and that we should have respect for ourselves and each other. Although it is often confused with aggression, nothing could be further from the truth. Aggressive, passive and manipulative behaviour are all examples of behaviour that is not assertive. Assertiveness involves the following:

- Knowing your own needs;
- Having respect for yourself;
- Having respect for others;
- Being open and honest whenever appropriate;
- Being able to compromise.

Becoming more assertive involves raising an awareness of how current behaviour may be contributing to relationship and other problems, and learning strategies to overcome this. For example, people learn ways of saying 'no', how to speak up for themselves, and how to give and receive criticism. All of this does not happen overnight; assertiveness courses can be lengthy. However, in this context, the issue can be adequately addressed by providing patients with a well-compiled summary, along with the suggestion that they can take a full course or read a book on the subject if they think it would be of benefit.

Here are two fairly typical examples:

Case history 4.2

Betty had one daughter and two grandchildren, of whom she was very fond. Although she had a part-time job in the grocer's shop, which tired her out, she loved to look after the two girls, who were aged 4 and 7, for her daughter whenever she could. Recently, her daughter has been taking her for granted, assuming she will take care of the girls, often with no notice and even if she has other plans, and she just cannot say no to her. Betty also does shopping and housework for an elderly neighbour, even though he has family of his own. Recently, she has been feeling completely drained, very tense, and starts at the slightest noise. She just cannot seem to relax, and has developed neck and shoulder pain.

Case history 4.3

Ali works in a large high street shop and has just been promoted to supervise a number of sales assistants. He is finding it stressful because none of the assistants like him, and they seem to go out of their way to annoy him. He feels depressed and cannot think what he has done to upset them. He thinks it might have something to do with how he deals with them if they need to be told about something they are doing wrong. He just seems to make them angry because he finds it difficult to criticize in a way that does not devalue them.

Betty just cannot say 'no', and needs to learn how to do so in a way that other people can accept. She will then take control of her work-load, and be able to tailor it to her abilities. If Ali can learn how to criticize constructively and with courtesy, his colleagues will begin to respect him and he will enjoy his work again.

Cushioning from the effects of stress

In many cases, where little or nothing can be done about the stress itself, the only solution is to cushion the patient from its effects. Even if something can be done about the stress, this is likely to take some time, so cushioning will calm a sensitized nervous system while changes are put into place.

Relaxing the mind and body

The arousal and resulting muscle tension brought about by stress can be very persistent and difficult to relieve. For many patients, the straight-forward answer to this is to spend time regularly on an activity that reduces arousal and tension in the muscles. Most individuals would find it relatively easy to identify a suitable activity: a warm lazy bath, listening to a favourite piece of music, aromatherapy, a walk on the beach, yoga, gardening, sport and so on. The choice of activity is very much down to personal taste and effectiveness.

However, particularly for chronic stress, there can be several draw-backs to this approach:

- Arousal and tension may be so persistent that the muscles need to be relaxed frequently, several times a day or more.
- The patient may be so tense, that this kind of approach just does not work.
- Arousal and tension often occur while doing something else, such as while in the workplace.
- An individual may not be able to find an everyday activity that encourages relaxation.
- Most of these activities are very time consuming.

In all of these scenarios, relaxation exercises are the simplest and most convenient substitute. The idea of these exercises dates back to 1938, when Jacobson introduced progressive relaxation, which is effective even for severe tension. He developed a method that demon-strated that if a muscle is first tensed, it will then automatically relax. The patient would progressively tense then relax each muscle group in turn, until the whole body was relaxed and arousal reduced. Regular practice was required to acquire the skill.

Since then, methods of relaxing without first tensing the muscles have been developed, including techniques to relax the mind as well as the body. With practice, these techniques can be used quickly and effectively in almost any situation. Patients who work can use the shorter techniques at lunch-time, or during coffee-breaks, or even whilst working, with longer sessions saved for later on at home. Instructions for these can be provided in written, audio or video form as appropriate. Carlson and Hoyle (1993) found relaxation training to be most effective if given individually, and also if the patient is given an audiotape of instructions to use at home.

Biofeedback techniques have also been introduced. These involve giving the patient auditory or visual feedback on their reducing tension and arousal level, which encourages the process of relaxation to

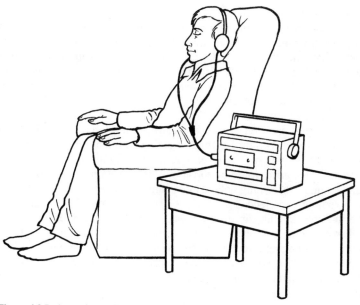

Figure 4.2 Patient using audio cassette for relaxation.

continue. Many patients particularly enjoy this method, and enjoy watching the pointer fall or the sound level reduce on the particular equipment they are using. High street shops now have such devices available at quite a reasonable cost.

With practice, many of these techniques can achieve relaxation in as little as a few minutes or, in some subjects, even more quickly. Patients can therefore try out a range of these relaxation techniques, to find which one, for them, is the most practical, enjoyable and effective. Whichever technique they choose, it should be used regularly, at first to acquire the skill, then to cushion the effects of stress by reducing and inhibiting arousal.

Almost everyone can use relaxation techniques, but Stephen Palmer of the London Centre for Stress Management suggested in 1992 that care should be exercised with certain patients. Those for whom the initial increase in blood pressure or muscle tension brought about by tensing the muscles might be dangerous should not use the methods that involve this process. In addition, there is a small minority of patients, usually those with an anxiety disorder, who may actually have a panic attack when using techniques involving relaxation or breathing exercises.

Breathing techniques

As we have seen, one of the most comon outcomes of stress is chronic hyperventilation, a condition that can insidiously undermine normal body function and produce a wide range of the symptoms associated with stress. Doctors will also be familiar with patients who are frightened by these symptoms, and fear major illness. As already suggested, setting their minds at rest on this score is all part of managing their stress problem.

All doctors are well versed in treating acute hyperventilation, but they may be less familiar with treating chronic low-level hyper-ventilation. This is best relieved through the regular use of breathing exercises designed to re-establish normal breathing rhythms. Slow diaphragmatic breathing not only does this but, by encouraging the type of breathing experienced in sleep, it also has a very calming effect on the individual. This can even be used instead of relaxation exercises. Other breathing exercises aim to introduce normal breathing patterns with a less calming effect; these can be used when the individual needs to remain alert. A simple and effective breathing exercise is included in the text for a patient booklet in Appendix 5.

Lifestyle changes

The fact has already been established that the lifestyle changes that people tend to make in times of stress often make matters worse. As stress management has developed, many suggestions for lifestyle changes that do cushion the effects of stress have been put forward and found to be effective. Once again, individuals have to assess these on the basis of their particular stress, and choose which ones they can incorporate into their lives.

Making too many changes at once is to be discouraged, and patients should take on only one change at a time, using a simple diary to monitor their progress and plan their next step. Attempting too many changes at once is not only likely to fail for practical and motivational reasons, but can produce further stress, since change itself is stressful. Fitting in a game of golf, making time for breakfast every day, and cutting down on coffee can seem easy and a novelty for one week, or even two, but then life can quickly get in the way and the new-found lifestyle will quickly slip away. Finding half an hour to kick a ball about with the family, a couple of times a week to begin with, can be both enjoyable and easy to sustain in the long term. Further changes can then be built on this firm foundation, over a period of time.

Here are some of the main strategies for stress management that are associated with the following aspects of everyday life:

- *Eating* Eating a well-balanced diet should of course be encouraged, but eating for comfort must be avoided. Regular meals, especially breakfast and lunch, are important in maintaining constant and appropriate blood sugar levels. Coffee and other drinks or foods containing caffeine should be avoided, as they simply increase arousal.

- *Time management* Taking regular breaks from a stressful situation is very important, as this allows arousal to be reduced regularly, and will gradually diminish the overall sensitivity of the nervous system. This principal operates at several levels. A 10-minute break every morning, a day out at the weekend, or two weeks on holiday in the summer all help to inhibit stress. Other strategies include being organized, keeping lists and a diary, planning ahead, prioritizing, delegating, setting realistic goals, and so on.
- *Leisure* Hobbies and pastimes provide an excellent cushion against stress, by reducing arousal, or providing an outlet for it, and by giving a break. They also help to prevent an individual's identity and self-image hinging entirely on the stressful situation.
- *Exercise* There is growing evidence that regular exercise can moderate the stress response, and even reduce depression and anxiety. It can also provide an outlet for physical arousal.
- *Sleep* Getting enough quality sleep is essential.
- *Substance use* The use of alcohol, tobacco or nonprescription drugs to alleviate stress is not recommended at all.

Making use of a support network
Those with little social support are vulnerable to stress, and will find that coping with daily hassles and the stresses of life is especially difficult. Doctors will all have lonely patients for whom they themselves may be the only source of support, but lonely people living alone are not the only individuals who might lack social support. Anyone living in a family or neighbourhood that does not provide this support is vulnerable. Many patients may even be the victims of negative social support, for example a spouse who is openly critical and non-supportive. For all of these patients, the role of the GP is particularly crucial.

Those patients who already have a support system should be encouraged to make maximum use of it as an outlet for feelings and as a source of encouragement. They can also accept offers of help and delegate to others to relieve pressure. Those without support should actively be encouraged to build their own, one step at a time, by creating new relationships and involvement in the community, or by seeking support from an appropriate community organization.

Changing how the person sees the situation

Thinking habits and beliefs

> There is nothing either good or bad, but thinking makes it so.
>
> (William Shakespeare, 1564–1616)

We all know people who remain positive and uncowed in the face of difficult circumstances, and others who simply crumple and give up hope. The difference lies purely in how these individuals think about their situation. Our thinking is not fixed for life; it can be changed.

Changing how we think about the world may make little difference to our stress if we are bereaved or in an abusive relationship, but we have already shown how, in the grey areas of stress, our appraisal of the situation can have a major impact on whether we experience stress or not. How we think about the world can even be a significant cause of stress in the first place. We are not considering pathological thinking here, simply normal everyday patterns of thought and belief that encourage and exacerbate stress in the modern world. This fabric of belief and thought has been woven from our childhood and life experiences, and is probably significantly coloured by our cultural background.

There have been many developments in this area since the 1960s. These have given rise to a range of methods by which individuals may alter their thinking in ways that can reduce stress. The linking theme is first to make individuals aware of the thinking styles and beliefs that may be causing problems, and then to make suggestions on how these might be changed. For many individuals, simply becoming aware of their established patterns of thought, along with their effects, can be enough to produce a substantial, efficacious and long-lasting change.

To anyone not familiar with such techniques, they may seem unusual and even strange, perhaps reminiscent of Tony Hancock in the 1960s repeating into his mirror, 'Every day in every way, I am getting better and better.' Even more strange is the fact that most patients, even those who do not have difficulty with stress, find the following ideas fascinating, enlightening and even liberating. They also find these techniques surprisingly effective.

Challenging irrational beliefs

In 1962, Albert Ellis began to explain how stress can be the outcome of beliefs about the world held by an individual. He described these as irrational beliefs in the sense that they are inflexible and dogmatic. Such beliefs are entirely nonpathological and extremely common. Here are a few taken from an extensive list of examples; it is easy to see how holding just one of these beliefs can make life stressful even in the absence of major negative life events:

- Life should be fair.
- I should be able to do everything well.
- There should be a perfect solution for everything.
- I need everyone's approval for nearly everything I do.
- I should not make a mistake.

Most of this thinking arises from growing up and living in a world where performance standards are set high, praise for a job well done is seen as encouraging an undesirable swollen head, and criticism of mistakes is never far away. All of this has produced low self-esteem and fear of failure in many people. If patients can become aware of and challenge these beliefs, their capacity for stress should be reduced.

Most of these beliefs are therefore not undisputed truth, but have their roots in childhood and the culture around us. Patients should be encouraged to ask themselves where these beliefs are written down or stated. Here are the same set of irrational or mistaken beliefs, along with ways of challenging them in parenthesis:

- Life should be fair. (Who says so? How could it be?)
- I should be able to do everything well. (Who says so? Do you know anyone else who can?)
- There should be a perfect solution for everything. (Who says so? How could there be?)
- I need everyone's approval for nearly everything I do. (Why? Who says so? Is it possible anyway? You cannot please all the people all the time.)
- I should not make a mistake. (Do you know anyone who does not make lots of them?)

Many common stress-inducing beliefs include the words 'ought', 'should' or 'must', the use of the latter often being described as 'musterbation':

- I ought to have done that better. (Why? Who says so?)
- I must cope with everything. (Why? Who says so?)
- I should have done that better. (Why? Who says so?)
- I must not make a mistake. (Everyone does; why not you?)
- I must get all this done today. (Why? Who says so?)

Other beliefs and thoughts involve the words 'awful', 'terrible' or 'can't stand it', which usually exaggerate the reality of the situation:

- I can't stand this. (You have stood things like this before. You can do it again. Is it really as bad as all that?)

- This is absolutely awful/terrible. (Some things are, but is this? What words have you left to use if something even worse happens?)

Case history 4.4

Wendy has consulted her GP because she feels depressed and stressed all the time. She cannot think of any reason for this as she has a nice house, two well-adjusted children and a good relationship with her husband. When asked to describe her usual day, she says,

> I must get the shopping and housework done before lunch-time, so that I can get to work on time at one o'clock. I must leave the house tidy. I have this absolutely awful job at the supermarket, stacking shelves. I can't stand it, but we need the money. Then I rush home to cook dinner. I really ought to do more home cooking and baking for the family but trying to fit everything in is so terribly difficult. It isn't fair really, I try so hard, but I never seem to get it right. There must be some easy answer to it all, because everybody else seems to cope better than I do.

Much of Wendy's thinking is causing her unnecessary stress. She sets rules and expectations for herself that are impossible to meet, exaggerates situations, and is angry with life because it does not all work out the way she wants. It is quite common for much of this type of thinking to interlock together in a kind of ideology of life. It is not being suggested that Wendy deliberately thinks in this way. These are thinking habits and beliefs that can creep up on people in today's hectic world where success and coping are so valued. It is therefore very common indeed.

So extensive is the possible range of irrational thinking that Ellis and his colleague Robert Harper (1975) were able to complete an entire book on the subject, called *A New Guide to Rational Living*. Detailed therapy focusing on this concept is called rational emotive therapy. However, stress management advice can restrict itself to pointing out some of the main areas and types of irrational thinking and their effects. Experience has shown that this can have a striking and rapid effect on patients.

Thinking more positively

In addition to his plan for stress inoculation training, Donald Meichenbaum has developed stress management techniques based on the idea that our self-speech (the constant inner dialogue we have with ourselves) exerts considerable control over our behaviour. Patients may therefore have a very negative and self-defeating style of self-speech, which compounds an already low self-esteem. This again is a common outcome of today's society and might include thoughts such as :

- This is going to be really difficult, I do not think I can cope with it.

- I will never manage this.
- I am hopeless at this.
- Oh no, here we go again.

This inner speech is therefore seen as a habit that can be changed, so the patient is made aware of this and encouraged to use other phrases, such as:

- I have coped with this before, so I can do it again.
- I know I can do this if I try.
- I know I can do this quite well, and that should be good enough.

Gaining a sense of control
Control is a theme that has run through much of the discussion of stress thus far, and we return to it here. We saw how people vary in the extent to which they feel they can affect their situation, and have some control over what happens to them (see Case history 3.5). Those with what was described as an external locus of control feel that they have very little control, and may be appraising their situation inappropriately and have taken none of the available steps to reduce their stress. Stress management is, in general, about empowering people and enabling them to deal with their difficulties effectively; this is particularly true in such cases. We have seen that there are many situations over which people really do have little control but, whenever it is possible, patients who feel they can do nothing to affect their situation require encouragement to change their minds and take action.

This idea may lie at the heart of the difference between people who crumple and those who flourish when faced with adversity. The former see the situation as beyond their control and give up, whilst the latter take control and put into place the required action to turn the situation around.

Tackling workplace stress

Workplace stress is just the same as any other stress in that all the techniques just given should be considered, and those that are relevant selected for use. In a moment we will think this through in a little more detail by looking at the four main areas that have just been discussed. However, the employer probably bears the major responsibility for stress in their workforce, and many organizations are now beginning to take this on board. How they are tackling this will also be considered shortly.

Before discussing what the individuals and organizations can do, it cannot be emphasized enough that great care and thought must be taken before a patient decides to tackle the problem head-on at work. Suddenly trying out new assertiveness skills on the boss can endanger a job. Even just admitting to stress can risk a current job or future prospects.

What individuals can do for themselves

The first thing someone suffering from stress in the workplace would be asked to do is to work through a list of the causes of this type of stress, such as the one given in Chapter 2, and tick off which of these are causing the problem. It is difficult to generalize with so many different scenarios for workplace stress, but let us go back through the four main areas, and see how these might be applied by the patient. As shown in Figure 4.3, we shall do this in a different order to that followed in the chapter so far, as this will prove more illuminating for workplace stress.

Providing information and explanation about stress
This will apply just as much in workplace stress as in any other.

Changing how the person sees the situation
As we saw, this can be the source of the problem in the first place. It may also be making a minor stress that could be coped with into a major one that cannot. Using their checklist, patients should assess whether their thinking has any bearing on each item causing stress. If they think it has, they should begin working on changing their thinking to reduce the stress, and also move on to consider the next area, and how they might resolve the cause of the stress. If they do not think that their thinking style is contributing to their stress, they should move straight on to consider the next area (resolving the cause).

Resolving the cause of the stress
The next thing that patients should now consider is the overall picture of their stress, and think through these three steps:

• *Step 1* Are they a square peg in a round hole? Is their personality really not suited to the job? If this is so, and they are to able to change their job, the problem is solved. If there is a mismatch, but they cannot change the job, they should move onto the next area (cushioning).

• *Step 2* Do they have a low tolerance for stress? If so, can they find a less stressful job? If not, cushioning is again the best solution.

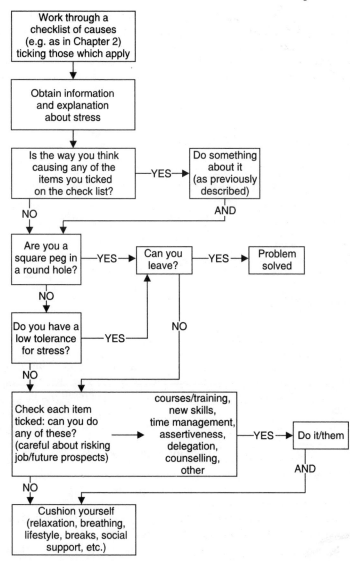

Figure 4.3 Tackling workplace stress.

- *Step 3* Using their check list, for each item ticked, patients should decide whether and how each cause of stress might be resolved. Are they assertive enough? Do they lack other skills? Will trying to do something about the problem put their job or their future at risk?

They should also decide whether any of the following would make a difference and, if so, decide whether to find out more about them:
- Assertiveness;
- Confidence building;
- Time management;
- Delegation;
- Taking breaks;
- Learning more about new skills and new technology;
- Counselling at work.

Again, if, having worked through the list, either nothing can be done or the patient chooses to do nothing, then cushioning is the best option.

As we shall see shortly, some employers already provide a range of training and counselling, and many others are thinking about it. This provision is likely to expand, particularly in the wake of the recent case of a social worker having successfully sued his employer for damages due to stress at work. If, however, the patient decides it is prudent to take no direct action on his or her work stress, the only answer is to cushion its effects.

Cushioning the effects of stress

Cushioning patients from their work stress is often the only solution if either the way of thinking about the situation cannot be changed, or nothing can be done to change the situation itself. GPs will have noticed that this is an increasingly common scenario that is presenting itself in primary care.

What the employer should do to manage workforce stress

With the increase in work stress and legal actions against them, American companies are beginning to provide stress prevention training and counselling for their workforces. Europe and the UK have been slow to follow suit, with only a few companies making such provision. According to the Health and Safety at Work Act of 1974, employers must ensure that their workplace is safe and healthy. This includes ensuring that there is no risk to health due to excessive and sustained levels of stress. In 1995, The Health and Safety Executive produced a book, *Stress at Work: a Guide for Employers*, in which they explain how employers should tackle the problem.

According to Cooper *et al.* (1988), organizations require to approach stress at three levels:

- Carry out a stress audit to establish the sources of stress arising from the working environment, how work is organized, how people deal with each other at work, and the day-to-day demands placed upon the workforce;
- Establish stress management programmes;
- Establish a counselling service.

Roslyn Taylor also suggested at a CBI conference in 1992 that there are positive benefits from providing some or all of the following skills training, depending on the outcome of the stress audit. This is very much in accord with our discussion so far about the sorts of reasons for workplace stress:

- Stress management;
- Relaxation;
- Time management;
- Assertiveness;
- Team building;
- Interpersonal skills;
- Management skills.

The Scottish Association for Mental Health produced a report (Devitt, 1994) by a working group that had examined the provision made by 146 companies and organizations. Just over one third had some form of support for staff with personal problems including stress. Some, such as British Telecom, had in-house counselling, whilst others, such as BBC Scotland, had bought in this service. Marks and Spencer had trained their own managers and supervisors to provide counselling. The working group concluded that the essential features of such a scheme included:

- Total confidentiality;
- Good awareness of the scheme amongst employees;
- Management personnel trained to recognize the signs that a problem may be developing;
- Good, experienced and impartial counsellors;
- Counselling separate from disciplinary procedures.

Unfortunately, for most employers, a full stress audit and a counselling service are very expensive options so, in practice, if anything at all, the more inexpensive option of providing stress management training for staff is most likely to be provided.

Summary

- GPs cannot remove stress from today's society; they can only treat its victims.
- Knowing how to recognize and deal with stress does not come naturally to people.
- Doctors do not need a detailed knowledge of stress management to make use of it with their patients.
- There are four main aspects to stress management:
  - Providing information and explanation, especially about symptoms;
  - Resolving the cause of stress, for example by becoming more assertive;
  - Cushioning the effects of stress by relaxation and breathing exercises, lifestyle changes and making use of social support;
  - Changing how the patient sees the situation, by becoming aware of thinking habits and beliefs that can create stress.
- Employers are increasingly recognizing the problem, and offering stress management or counselling to employees.

Part Two

Stress and the General Practitioner

5

The physiology and psychology of stress

GPs are frequently involved in the treatment of stress in one way or another. It is part of modern life and so it impinges upon the GP's practice of medicine. Medical students are not taught a great deal about the management of stress; new entrants to general practice can therefore find it a difficult condition to treat. Yet, with a little knowledge and expertise, stress is an interesting and rewarding field, with treatment being both practical and successful.

Treating stress is an exercise in applied psychology and applied physiology. These two subject areas are interrelated and some knowledge of both is essential if a doctor is to treat patients adequately. It is the unique nature of the diagnosis and treatment of stress that makes it so interesting to study and so rewarding to treat. Doctors are used to treating medical conditions that have an established pathology, histology and physical signs, and a rational treatment that may include medication or surgery or other related therapeutic options. Conditions that lie outwith these parameters are described in medical school as being 'functional' and are largely ignored.

P. G. F. Nixon, a consultant cardiologist at the Charing Cross Hospital, has addressed these problems over many years and summarizes them in a chapter in a book entitled *Changing Ideas in Health Care*, (Nixon, 1989). He gives an account of the physiology of stress in relation to the rehabilitation of patients who have suffered myocardial infarction, but there are also general applications.

The GP registrar will find, upon entering general practice, that there is an abundance of patients suffering from this type of nonspecific condition. This can be disturbing because there does not seem to be a rationale to the varied presenting complaints. Without a rational diagnostic protocol, new entrants to general practice can sometimes feel at a loss when it comes to establishing a diagnosis and recommending treatment. Is there a rational pathology that unites these apparently dissociated conditions? We will next consider three patients with apparently disparate conditions.

Stressed patients: various presentations

Case history 5.1

Mrs A. C. is a married woman, aged 35 years. She sits down warily, but makes easy eye contact and appears active and agitated. She volunteers information regarding her complaint without prompting, explaining that she is tired all the time. She is totally exhausted, goes to bed early, sometimes at nine o'clock, and sleeps like a log all night, but this does not stop her from feeling so very tired. Things have got so bad that she can no longer cope and something will have to be done because something is clearly wrong. Her tiredness has become the most important thing in her life, taking over everything. Her manner is pejorative and it almost seems as if she thinks that the doctor is responsible for her tiredness.

Case history 5.2

Mr D. R. is aged 29 years, unmarried but in a stable relationship. He sits down cautiously and explains quietly that his problem is of a personal nature. He avoids eye contact and is not sure where to start, but eventually admits to a bladder problem. It has been present for many months, but it is getting worse and he now has some difficulty in managing it. He finds that after he has passed water he has difficulty controlling the stream, tending to dribble a bit, but, after he has left the toilet, he can develop an intense irritation deep between his legs, which can be unbearable. Sometimes he will involuntarily pass a few more drops of urine, which is very distressing. When this occurs, the irritation stops. Sometimes the irritation goes on for hours and he feels that he cannot stand it for much longer. He admits to being stressed and has had difficulty with concentrating and sleeping. The relationship between him and his partner is deteriorating.

Case history 5.3

Miss T. K. is aged 24 years and soon to be married. She admits that she is not coping very well with life, and is extremely worried about her coming marriage, as she is not sure that it is the right thing to do. She feels that she is under a lot of parental pressure to marry her boyfriend, but she herself is not sure. She is losing sleep and has been warned at her work. She is also suffering from abdominal cramps and her abdomen is often grossly swollen so that she is unable to wear her old skirts. She sometimes has diarrhoea, but on other occasions she is constipated.

We can assume for the purposes of this book that all of these patients are stressed, although it might be necessary to perform some investigations in order to establish this fact by excluding other conditions.

A unifying pathology

If these three apparently different conditions have a unifying pathology, they have to be considered as a single disease process. The first patient is tired all the time, the second is suffering from pseudoprostatism, and the third has an irritable bowel syndrome. These are all established conditions and they can all be associated with stress. How can stress produce so many different symptoms?

An understanding of the disease process requires a knowledge of basic physiology because stress-related conditions are caused by a disorder of normal physiology. Physiology is changed by stress and the way that this happens is best illustrated by the arousal curve, which plots arousal against performance, as shown in Figure 5.1.

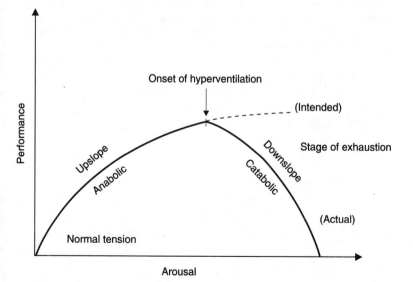

Figure 5.1 The arousal curve. (After P. G. F. Nixon, 1989.)

The arousal curve

Performance is defined as the ability of an individual to cope and adapt. Arousal is defined as the general drive state of the individual or the level of effort and distress.

The physiological implications of the arousal curve explain many of the observed clinical phenomena related to stress. In the curve arousal, which is related to stress, initially increases our ability to perform tasks. Arousal increases performance, but only up to a point. There comes a time at which increasing arousal fails to improve performance and then starts to diminish it. This is the downslope and it is there that symptoms start to occur.

It can be seen that on the first part of the arousal curve the individual begins to respond to the stress or challenge with an increase in sympathetic activity and anabolic hormones predominate. When the downslope occurs, the pituitary/adrenocortical response predominates and catabolic steroids are released. There is a catabolic shift and it is this event that begins to produce chronic symptoms. The symptoms of stress are due to sympathetic overactivity and adrenal cortex overstimulation and can be psychological as well as physical; they include emotionalism, tearfulness, loss of concentration, feelings of worthlessness and altered behaviour.

This catabolic shift also produces physical symptoms (which appear logical when one considers the hormonal changes that occur), together with other changes taking place at the commencement of the downslope (e.g. rises in plasma levels of cholesterol and low density lipids) (Sterling and Eyer, 1988):

- Anabolic hormones are released during sympathetic activity on the first part of the arousal curve, where they predominate:
  - Insulin;
  - Calcitonin;
  - Testosterone;
  - Oestrogen;
  - Prolactin;
  - Luteinizing hormone;
  - Follicle stimulating hormone;
  - Gonadotrophin releasing hormone;
  - Prolactin releasing hormone;
  - Atriopeptin;
  - Thymosins;
  - Lipokinase;
  - Cytokinase.

- Catabolic hormones increase when the arousal curve passes the physiological tolerance point:
  - Glucocorticoids;
  - Epinephrine;
  - Growth hormone;
  - Glucagon;
  - Antidiuretic hormone;
  - Renin;
  - Angiotensin;
  - Aldosterone;
  - Erythropoietin;
  - Thyroxine;
  - Parathormone;
  - Melatonin;
  - Thyroid releasing hormone;
  - Adrenocorticotrophic hormone;
  - Encephalin;
  - Dynorphin;
  - Entrophin.

Inappropriate breathing

In many ways, the most significant change that occurs at the point of maximum physiological tolerance is the onset of inappropriate breathing. This was studied and explained by L. C. Lum of the Respiratory Physiology Unit of Papworth and Addenbrooks Hospital in 1977. By inappropriate breathing is meant hyperventilation, an increase in the tidal volume due to a preponderance of thoracic respiration and increased sighing.

Normal respiration is mainly abdominal, with little effort being contributed by the muscles of the thorax. It is even, quiet and unobtrusive. When a stressed individual has passed the point of maximum tolerance described by Nixon (1989), respiration changes to that described by Lum, which is illustrated by the traces of respiratory movements shown in Figure 5.2 (see pages 76 and 77).

The physiological outcome of this maladaptive breathing is of great significance. It eliminates an excess amount of carbon dioxide, producing a respiratory alkalosis due to the loss of carbonic acid, so that the body excretes alkalis in an effort to maintain the normal pH. When the alkaline buffering mechanisms become depleted, the patient is forced to hyperventilate in order to avoid acidotic shifts. Lactic acid cannot be buffered after exertion and so builds up *in situ*, causing

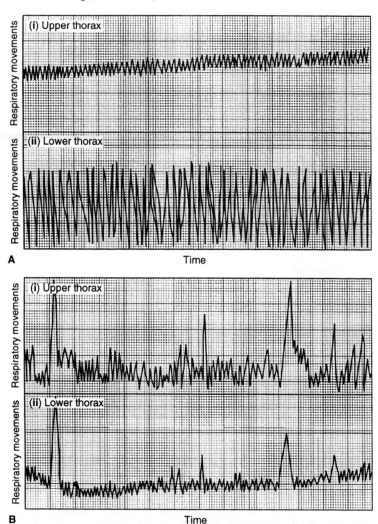

Figure 5.2 Traces of respiratory movements. **A**: Normal respiratory movements in a 57-year-old male, showing: (**i**) relatively slight movements of the upper thorax, and (**ii**) a preponderance of diaphragmatic excursions of the lower thorax. **B**: Respiratory movements of a 26-year-old agoraphobic female, demonstrating hyperventilation. Note (**i**) the preponderance of upper thoracic excursions, with (**ii**) the relatively slight use of the diaphragm as shown in the lower thorax recording, and also the grossly irregular pattern and sighs (indicated by tall spikes). **C**: Respiratory movements of a 39-year-old male with pseudoangina, demonstrating hyperventilation. Note the increased use of the upper thorax (**i**), the gross irregularity and frequent sighs. (Redrawn from original electronic recordings made by L. C. Lum, 1977.)

painful muscles. When lactic acid reaches the pH monitoring centres in the brain, compensatory overbreathing is induced. This typically occurs in the early morning, waking the patient. Stress-related disorders can thus be mistaken for a depressive illness.

Inhalational anaesthesia has always been considered safe because of its immediate reversibility. Respiratory control of acid/base buffering should be constantly changing, but maladaptive respiration is constant and the changes in blood acidity are constant. Nixon points out that attempting to relax can produce hypocapnia, which has an adrenergic effect, producing anxiety and somatic symptoms which further stimulate hyperventilation. It also produces hypersensitivity to stimuli and hyperactivity.

This chronic hyperventilation syndrome was well described by Bernard Lewis in 1959, when he published a study of 250 patients with chronic hyperventilation problems. He was able to demonstrate that cardiac adaptability to hyperventilation is significantly worse in patients who habitually overbreathe than it is in controls. Such patients also have a range of other stress-related symptoms.

Other factors

Nixon (1989) also showed that sympathetic/parasympathetic imbalance occurs, and that high levels of arousal create a diuresis of magnesium

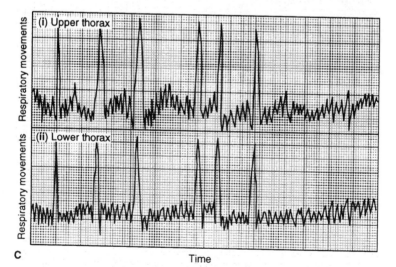

Figure 5.2 *Continued*

which has similar effects to a calcium channel blocker, causing the muscular tubes of the body to constrict. This is of particular importance in the generation of symptoms. Many patients suffering from stress have seemingly diverse and obscure symptoms and syndromes caused by this effect. Many disease processes that are assumed to be stress-related, conditions such as dysmenorrhoea, irritable bowel syndrome or psuedoprostatism, can be explained by the phenomenon of smooth muscle excitability and contractibility, causing dysfunction of visceral tubular structures.

The clinical case histories

It is in the light of these findings that the three clinical presentations introduced earlier can be considered. The multiplicity of possible symptomatology defies imagination. Diagnosis and treatment would be impossible if it were not for the fact that some of the symptoms experienced by stressed patients are almost universally present. Using our knowledge of the physiology involved, it is possible to consider the three patients mentioned, who are typical of the stressed patients so frequently seen in general practice. Understanding the disease process is essential to the understanding of the treatment proposed.

Explanation of symptoms

Three syndromes are presented. The first patient is tired all the time; she has a chronic fatigue syndrome. The second patient has chronic pseudoprostatism and the third has an irritable bowel syndrome. They all have differing degrees of awareness of the nature of their problems. It is very clear, however, that they have a unifying pathology: they are all stressed. They have all passed their point of maximum physiological tolerance.

The first patient is not achieving restoring sleep. She has a build-up of lactic acid in her tissues by day, producing muscle pain so that her muscles are stiff and sore and she has little tolerance of exercise. During sleep the lactic acid is recycled and her sleep pattern is disturbed, so that she wakes up in the morning feeling tired with a painful neck, jaw and shoulders, something she will admit to on direct questioning. The briefest consideration of the possible changes in her physiological state on the downslope would explain why she might feel unwell in other ways.

The second patient, the young man, suffers from pseudoprostatism. He is experiencing urethral spasm triggered by micturition. The urethra constricts, trapping urine in the proximal urethra at the bulbous muscles. The presence of this urine is extremely uncomfortable and creates further spasm. In extreme cases, this discomfort can become a severe pain and the patient can be virtually disabled. On direct questioning, the patient will admit to other symptoms because, as is obvious from the pathology, stress-related symptoms are unlikely to exist in isolation. This patient has a predominating symptom. He will also have neck and shoulder pain and other symptoms.

The last patient has an irritable bowel syndrome with intestinal colic. Again, this is a hollow viscus problem with peristaltic dysfunction. It might be due to magnesium depletion due to dysfunctional breathing or hormonal influences, but, as far as the GP is concerned, it is enough to understand that there is a rational pathology and that rational treatment is possible for all three of these patients.

Psychological implications

It is important not to ignore the psychological implications of these physiological phenomena. Indeed, the physiology has not been fully explained in this text. The role of the hypothalamus and the hypothalamic/pituitary neurological and portal systems is of importance in a study of the minutiae of stress responses, and has been the subject of much study, as has the hippocampus. The results are too detailed to be reported here. The impact of cognitive and emotional factors is thus possible via the hypothalamus before the development of physiological symptoms and may be the initiating cause. The severity of the symptoms and the patient's inability to cope can produce psychological symptoms such as anxiety or depression. To complicate the situation further, the symptoms experienced by a stressed person are the same as those that one would expect in an individual who is anxious for understandable exogenous reasons. The patient who feels anxious, then, has a long feed-back loop to the hypothalamus, which makes the symptoms worse.

Autonomic arousal during individual tasks

Hardy and Heyes (1987) describe early work by Yerkes and Dodson, who, in 1908, looked at how a person's performance of a task varied according to their level of arousal. They found that there was an optimum level of arousal for each task, and that levels lower or higher than this reduced performance, as already shown in Figure 5.1. A medium level of arousal was therefore usually optimum. This means in today's terms that, when faced with an examination or a driving test, being either too relaxed or too stressed will reduce performance levels.

Yerkes and Dodson also found that this effect was more pronounced during complicated tasks, with performance dropping away quickly on either side of the optimum level of arousal. There may also be evidence to suggest that the optimum level of arousal may be greater for physical than for mental tasks, meaning, for example, that mental arithmetic is seriously affected by stress, whereas digging the garden may not be. Experience would probably bear this out. Extrapolating from this point, the 'fight or flight' reaction may simply be the extreme case of this process, wherein the highest level of arousal is actually the optimum required for the very physical task in hand.

Important work on the role of stress in preparing us to deal with environmental situations has also been carried out by the physician, Hans Seyle, who, in 1973, said, 'Everybody knows what stress is and nobody knows what it is.' In 1946 he described three stages in reacting to what he called environmental stressors. These stages formed a sequence which he called the general adaptation syndrome. These three stages were:

- Stage 1: Alarm reaction;
- Stage 2: Resistance;
- Stage 3: Exhaustion.

In stage one, the alarm reaction is provoked by any stressor and is adrenergic in character, as in the upslope of the arousal curve presented previously. These responses are maladaptive if there is no useful outlet for them.

In stage two, the stressor is resisted by the mobilized body and, if this is successfully achieved, there will be a return to equilibrium. If the resistance does not deal with the stressor, or if the stressor persists for too long, the third stage, that of exhaustion will be reached.

In stage three, which is synonymous with the downslope of the arousal curve, the alarm reaction reasserts itself, and the body's resources are depleted, leaving the body vulnerable to disease and dysfunction. This could be likened to the condition of depletion described today as 'burnout'.

Acute, chronic and intermittent stress

Seyle's concept of stress has practical implications for patients. Stress is not necessarily produced by the same type of stressor on every occasion and may be the result of acute, chronic, or even intermittent factors. A consideration of illustrative case histories may be helpful.

Case history 5.4

Jennifer is aged 45, single, and enjoys her own company in her small flat. Currently she has relatives staying with her from Canada, including two noisy small children. This week, she suddenly experienced a feeling of acute panic, palpitations, light-headedness and nausea whilst out shopping.

Case history 5.5

Gary has just taken his driving test and failed. He is aged 19 and was well prepared for the test, but he could not control his nerves on the day and made many silly mistakes.

Case history 5.6

Ethel has been caring for her elderly mother, who has senile dementia, in her own home for three years. She has no other family and feels it is her responsibility. She felt it to be stressful at first, but then seemed to become used to it, but, just recently, she feels drained and exhausted, and often feels her heart racing. She has also had several colds this winter.

Jennifer is clearly a patient who has experienced a panic attack as a result of the fight or flight response being triggered whilst thinking about her overcrowded flat; this is an acute problem. Her relatives will soon depart and hopefully all should be well again.

Gary has performed less well than he had hoped on his driving test because his arousal was too high, probably because the psychological threat of failure had invoked what Seyle called the alarm reaction. Here again is another case of acute stress.

Ethel has reached Seyle's third stage of adaptation, and is experiencing the unrelenting outcome of chronic stress, a potentially much more serious state of affairs.

Another factor that may contribute to the overall picture is intermittent stress, which can be just as damaging as chronic stress, if not more so.

Case history 5.7

James was made redundant from his job as a joiner. He applied for many other jobs and, after six months, was lucky to be offered a new position. While he was unemployed, he suffered from chest pain, which was diagnosed as being caused by stress, but this disappeared when he started his new job. Three months later, his wife had to have a major operation, leaving him to cope with two children on his own for several months. When she recovered, they managed to get away for a bit of a holiday, but, when they returned, their house had been burgled.

This sort of on–off stress can have serious effects on the patient. Not only is the person stressed whilst these events are going on, but they begin to anticipate the next thing that will go wrong, meaning that stress can persist long after the last situation that provoked it has disappeared.

Stress and anticipation

A common thread running through these and other case histories is the ability of human beings to anticipate and imagine the future. This unique ability lies at the heart of the modern experience of stress.

Gary can imagine what his friends will say if he fails his driving test; Jennifer can clearly picture the next weeks in her crowded flat; James is worried about what will go wrong next. People in general know exactly what their supervisor will say if that report is late again, when the next costly telephone bill is due, or what will happen if their teenage son moves on from an occasional ecstasy to a regular temazepam. These advanced cognitive abilities coexisting within a primitive body that still responds with ancient reflexes is a perfect formula for problems with stress.

Stresses accumulate

In view of our understanding of the physiology of stress, it is not surprising that the effect of a number of stressful situations is cumulative. One major problem can produce an equivalent effect to several medium difficulties or numerous small hassles. The daily hassles of life today can soon add up: the alarm did not go off, there was no milk left for breakfast, there was heavy traffic on the way to work, and then you realized you had forgotten to pick up a colleague on the way! Noisy neighbours, an argument with a partner, making this week's money last: everyone from every walk of life has their own set of daily hassles. This can reduce an individual's tolerance of additional stress.

One small extra problem can simply be the last straw, producing an arousal level that just cannot be handled. Many patients who consult their GPs who are suffering from the effects of stress may be completely baffled about the cause. The public perception is that there should be a serious, obvious and immediate cause for their difficulties, which is more than just their everyday hassles building up over time. Patients may be genuinely unaware of the cause of their stress and may deny that they are stressed.

Change is stressful

An important example of the cumulative effect of stress was suggested by the research of Holmes and Rahe (1967).

In general, arousal is low when the environment is stable and predictable. If any change occurs, whether for good or ill, we must adapt to that change, and arousal is produced. Building on Seyle's idea that continually having to adapt to life situations exerts a draining effect on the body, Holmes and Rahe therefore proposed that the more changes that a person has had to deal with over the previous one or two years, the lower was their resistance to disease. They developed a 'Life Events Survey', which listed some 43 events, with a score assigned to each. The death of a spouse and divorce were ranked the highest, with the celebration of Christmas, a minor violation of the law, or a vacation, being ranked the lowest.

The list also included retirement, moving house, getting married and changing job. The overall score indicated an individual's probable level of resistance and how likely that individual was to become ill because of the changes experienced. Indeed, Worden (1995), in reviewing the literature on bereavement, even suggests that the death of a spouse may be associated with a higher mortality rate for the survivor. This applied to both sexes, with the excess risk much greater for men.

Individual variation in response to stress

Eysenck (1967) suggested that there are individuals whose autonomic nervous system is called into action more easily than others. He suggested that variations in this lability of the autonomic nervous system produced a continuum of behaviour and experience for human beings, with very low lability producing a sense of stability, and high lability resulting in an experience of emotionality or stress in response to life events. Barlow (1988), in reviewing the evidence, suggests that this may in turn be due to labile neurotransmitter systems. This would mean that, for some people, it takes much less to induce a feeling of stress than for others. This is not a sign of weakness, as is often thought by patients; it is simply a sign of an individual biological difference, in the same way that height or eye colour may vary.

A labile nervous system would have been a positive advantage for our ancestors in terms of self-preservation, with such people able to deal far more quickly and effectively with a dangerous predator or other threat. It is only in the modern world that it becomes a problem. Eysenck even goes on to propose that the lability of the nervous system is likely to be inherited, with many animal studies demonstrating the ability to breed for certain emotional characteristics. Broadhurst (1958) has bred rats selectively for emotionality.

This variation in the nervous system also means that we experience differences in our need for stimulation. Mandler (1980) argues that we all need increases in general arousal, which he calls 'autonomic jags', and that it is this need that makes us want to change from one activity to another. Most people receive such 'jags' routinely in everyday life, but those with a very unresponsive nervous system find that they need to put themselves in very threatening or dangerous situations to experience this effect. Think of racing drivers, mountain climbers and other participants in dangerous sports, or live television presenters or performers, who explain their behaviour by saying that they need to do it to make them feel alive, or that they are 'hooked on adrenalin'.

Such people appear to thrive on stress, but, in reality, they are not truly stressed at all. Those at the other end of the spectrum, with a very reactive nervous system, can experience too much adrenergic excitement and become stressed very easily in response to life events. Luckily, most of us fit in somewhere between the two extremes.

Variation in the psychological response to stress

Added to these physiological differences there are psychological differences, which encourage or inhibit our vulnerability to stress. This powerful cocktail of individual differences means that there is tremendous variation in the aetiology of each patient's stress.

The 43 events listed by Holmes and Rahe, together with many others, are universally accepted as producing stress in those who experience them: bereavement, debt, overwork, serious illness, and so on. However, there are many situations and events that may cause stress in one person, but be seen as a bracing challenge, exciting, or even boring, by others. Public speaking, car racing, writing a report, amateur dramatics, abseiling, city driving or visiting the dentist are just a few examples. The difference must lie within the psychology of the individual.

There is a point at which the individual concerned has a vital role to play in deciding whether a situation is a threat or not. An important figure in introducing this idea was psychologist Richard Lazarus, whose seminal paper in 1952, with colleagues Deese and Osler, led the way to an understanding of the crucial, but unwitting, personal role of the individual in the production of his or her own stress. The central theme of this work was that the individual's appraisal of the situation will define whether stress is experienced or not. This appraisal will depend on the individual's personality and previous experience, thinking style and motivation.

Much work has since been done on this subject, looking at the personality variables and coping styles that make people more or less vulnerable to stress. This has been considered in detail separately in Chapter 3, but meanwhile consideration should be given to the crucial question of how the psychology and physiology of stress interact within an individual to exaggerate the problem.

Physiology and psychology: the interaction

An individual's physiology and psychology do not exist in isolation. They are interdependent and they inter-react in a complex way. They each stimulate the other and this has clinical implications.

Case history 5.8

Charles is the middle-aged manager of a busy chain store. The past six months have seen frequent changes in strategy and staffing in the store, and he has had to work late nearly every night. When he gets home he cannot relax, and is aware of his heart racing. This worries him so much that he is unable to sleep at night. He wakes feeling exhausted and tense and dreads going to work. Every day he seems to feel worse. Just recently he has noticed mild chest pain whilst at work, which has made him feel panicky. He is unable to put it off any longer and feels he must go to see his doctor; something serious must be wrong with his heart.

Here, the physical symptoms of stress produce anxiety in the affected individual. This in turn increases the stress response, producing more symptoms, and so on. A vicious circle has begun, with the patient becoming more and more anxious and stressed and fearing major organic illness. Similar fears can arise from many physical stress symptoms, especially those connected with headaches, the heart, breathing and balance.

Psychological symptoms can produce a similar, if not more frightening, effect for the patient.

Case history 5.9

Margaret is a single mother of three teenage boys, and has been divorced for three years. She is finding it hard to make ends meet, and finds coping with the family a strain. She often gets headaches, which feel as if a tight band is round her head, but she has also begun frequently to forget things, and finds the simplest decision a nightmare. She is very worried about this as her mother died of dementia, and she is afraid that these are the early signs. How on earth would the boys cope?

Case history 5.10

Melanie is being beaten by her boyfriend whenever he gets drunk, but he has threatened to come after her if she leaves him. If she goes to the shops, she feels strange, as if she is going to faint, and then she begins to be convinced she is about to lose control, break down and scream. She never actually does lose control, but she is convinced that she is going mad, and is afraid to tell anyone. It now happens every time she goes out.

These case histories again illustrate the powerful downward spiralling effect of the symptoms of stress feeding into the individual's psychology, and building on the fears, ignorance and stigma that exist there, to produce still more symptoms. The whole experience is distressing and disabling, and the GP is usually the first person to whom people will turn for help.

It can be seen from Figure 5.3 that the patient is caught in a cycle that generates anxiety. If the stress is not dealt with, things may get worse and worse because the cycle is self-perpetuating.

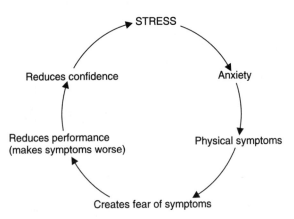

Figure 5.3 The anxiety cycle. (Redrawn from Hambly, 1991.)

Summary

- The response to stress is physical as well as psychological.
- Stress produces physiological changes.
- Stress produces psychological changes.
- Both changes create problems for the patient.
- Many common physical conditions can be explained by alterations in the patient's physiology.
- The response to stress is very individualistic.
- Problems may get worse if they are not addressed.

6

Management of the consultation

Patients suffering from stress-related conditions go to their doctor seeking treatment. What can the doctor do? What tools does the doctor have, and what knowledge? Treatment begins with the consultation which is the cornerstone of general practice and nowhere is it of more importance than in the management of stress-related disorders. The consultation can be the entire management cycle from beginning to end, it can be the first event in a referral process, or, of course, it can be unsuccessful in its treatment of the condition. Successful treatment requires good consultation skills and the co-operation of the patient. It requires an acceptance of the diagnosis by the patient and a contract or agreement between the doctor and the patient regarding treatment.

The doctor's attitude

Doctors will vary in the importance they place on stress in the aetiology of disease. Some doctors will see stress everywhere they look. Most ill patients will be stressed by their illness or perhaps incidentally. The majority of people experience stress in their lives at some time but most of them will cope with it without the need for medical intervention and do not see it as a medical condition. The same applies to some doctors, who will take the attitude that stress is not an illness and is not their problem.

Stress is one contributory factor of many in some conditions, so the frequency of the diagnosis of stress will vary from doctor to doctor. The ability or desire to identify a patient who may be stressed depends upon the attitude and approach of the doctor. Those who deny the existence of stress will never diagnose it and no doctor can diagnose a condition if he or she does not think of it in the first place.

There is great variation in the ways doctors conduct their con-sultations and their practices. Doctors practise in a way with which they are comfortable and which suits their personality and their approach to medicine. There is no place in medicine for the medical clone, so it would be inappropriate to suggest a proforma consultation for the stressed patient. None the less there are some hints and tips that may be of assistance to the new entrant to general practice, which may help in dealing with this type of problem.

This chapter relates to those patients whose primary diagnosis is stress or where stress is the principal problem underlying the symptoms with which the patient presents.

The presentation of stress: the patient's attitude

Each patient perceives his or her illness in a unique way, just as each patient experiences that illness in an individual way. No two patients are the same, and no two patients present the same illness in the same way. It would be advantageous to the doctor and greatly simplify treatment of the condition if each patient came in and stated that he or she was suffering from stress, that they had identified a stressor, and that they were experiencing certain physiological and psychological problems as a result. They could add that their work and their relationships were suffering because they were stressed. Patients do not often present in that way.

The aware patient

Some patients realize that they are stressed and attend with stress as their presenting complaint. They feel pressured and unable to cope. They may be short-tempered and aggressive. Sometimes it is their families who have asked them to come because of their behaviour, or they may know that their employers are unhappy with their performance at work. These patients know the cause of their stress but may be unable to do anything about it without guidance. They may have no unreal expectations regarding treatment and often say with a sigh: 'I know there's nothing you can do doctor. I'll have to sort it out myself.'

All GPs have patients like this and they are probably the easiest stressed patients to treat if they are prepared to co-operate in a management plan. They have insight and awareness and they may well co-operate because they are desperate for treatment by the time they reach the doctor's surgery. They may see their relationships, their jobs, their very lives unravelling before them and they know that something will have to be done.

The defended patient

A more common patient is the one who is not feeling well and not coping well, and at the same time is not prepared to admit that the problem is stress. Such patients can be of either sex and of any age or occupation. They make up a large proportion of the patients seen in general practice. Whether the GP identifies these patients as being stressed depends to some extent upon the personal philosophy of the doctor, but it is probably true that most modern vocationally trained GPs recognize the stressed patient and would prefer to treat the underlying cause of the problem than to treat the patient symptomatically.

Presenting symptoms

The symptoms that bring the patient to the doctor have been dealt with previously, as have their causes. There is no stereotyped patient. Patients can present with any combination of symptoms, possibly including some incidental symptoms unrelated to stress. If the patient is well defended or experiencing feelings of guilt, or has low personal esteem, and if that patient denies being stressed, diagnosis and treatment can be difficult. This, however, is a common presentation and this is a problem the doctor has to overcome.

The advantages of getting to the bottom of the patient's problem are clear. If the underlying condition is not adequately treated, the patient will not be helped, may return with different symptoms, and will be dissatisfied. The doctor may have to contend with an unhappy frequent attender, who may be sliding into a desperate social and personal situation. Stress-related problems can get worse. Not only does that patient suffer, so does his or her family and employer, and possibly a dependent relative, and, inevitably, so does the doctor. It is important that the doctor has the ability to identify and treat stress for these reasons, and also because the public are now informed about these matters and expect doctors to be competent in this area.

The consultation: the initial phase

When the patient enters the consulting room from the waiting room, that patient brings with himself or herself a certain amount of emotional and psychological baggage. They may have had to wait for some time in the waiting room and they will have used that time rehearsing what they will say to the doctor. The doctor of course will already have seen many patients, some difficult and some easy, but all of them demanding. It is not a good basis on which to start what may be a difficult consultation.

An American study has shown that the average doctor will interrupt the patient within 17 seconds of the start of the consultation. Thus the patient's rehearsed presentation will become disjointed and, although the object of the doctor's interruption is probably to accelerate the consultation, it may have the reverse effect. A good consultation will start with a welcome and an open-ended question, which will allow the patient free expression. Allowing the patient to pursue that free expression pays dividends. At the start of a consultation, both patient and doctor have particular problems.

The patient's problems

The patient may have attended unwillingly, and may feel that having to seek help is an admission of failure and that other people are able to cope with the problems that are now causing difficulty. As a result of these negative feelings, the patient may deny that he or she is stressed or that there are any stress-related problems at all.

A patient may be experiencing physical symptoms and may deny stress. There may be fear about the nature of these symptoms, a fear of diseases like cancer, or, if psychological symptoms predominate, there may be a fear of madness, which may or may not be expressed. There is usually a very real fear amongst patients that they will not be taken seriously, that they may be dismissed or perhaps humiliated, or that their problems will be described as being 'all in the mind'.

Patients may be apprehensive because they have no idea what to expect from the doctor, or worse, they may have unreal expectations about what can be achieved. Some will expect drug therapy, but some will resist drug therapy; very few will anticipate any form of constructive talking treatment. There may be hopelessness, doubts about their ability to help themselves, and inappropriate anger or resentment, some of which may eventually be directed at the doctor. Patients may also be depressed or anxious.

The doctor's problems

The doctor also has his or her emotional baggage. The last patient may have been depressed and the one before that also. It may be the end of a long surgery and the doctor may be prejudiced against stressed patients, or feel unable to cope with them adequately. There is always the pressure of time and the doctor may be painfully aware that there are four or five patients waiting. Doctors do not have the luxury of infinitely long consultations, even though patient survey after patient survey shows that what patients want most from doctors is time. Many doctors are also on call for emergencies as they consult, and may have a long list of pressing matters with which to deal. It is very difficult for a doctor in general practice to isolate the consultation from the rest of his or her daily obligations and concentrate on the individual patient, but stressed patients do need that investment of time and understanding.

The opening minutes

Consultations for stressed patients can be therapeutic for the patient and interesting for the doctor. If the patient is informed and aware, the consultation will be structured and productive. If the patient approaches the problem obliquely, it will take more time and will be less structured. The doctor should make allowances for the patient's fears and inhibitions and allow time for the patient to make his or her own case. Allowing time when the waiting room is full of irritable patients is not easy, but it pays dividends in the longer term.

Physical symptoms

A listening doctor using open and reflected questions will quite quickly form an impression of the patient's problems even though they may not be complaining of stress. The doctor may suspect that the underlying definitive diagnosis is stress, but that is not to say that the patient admits or acknowledges that diagnosis. A wise doctor will continue the consultation with care, cognizant of the patient's sensitivities.

Techniques appropriate to the consultation

The type of symptoms described and the demeanour of the patient are indicative of the aetiological role of stress if it is present. Further information can be obtained by using well-tried techniques appropriate to most consultations but which are particularly useful if the diagnosis is in doubt or if the consultation is going to be problematic. How do you start the interview? How do you progress it? An inexperienced doctor can have great difficulty in managing a demanding consultation, but that difficulty often springs from a perceived need to 'manage' the consultation actively: to have a beginning, a middle and an end, and to leave the consultation tidy.

Video-recordings of consultations show very quickly that very few follow this pattern. They tend to meander and to be unstructured with relevant information appearing at different times. Important information can appear and, because of the way it is presented, perhaps as a throwaway remark, it is missed by the doctor. It can be hard for the doctor to concentrate throughout a two-hour surgery and it may be that we ask too much of ourselves.

A consultation can always be managed if the doctor closes it down, if he or she sets the agenda and discourages expression and discussion. There is always a temptation to do that. There is an equal temptation to accept the patients's first presentation of the problem and deal with that, even if the doctor suspects that there is an alternative agenda that the patient really wishes to address. Successfully managing this type of consultation requires great skill and experience, and, of course, a desire on the part of the doctor to manage fully the patient's problems.

If the GP is going to be more than a mechanistic medical scientist, the doctor has to develop consultation skills. These skills have to be practised and rehearsed, but the rewards for so doing are great. The quality of consultations improves and more patients are treated successfully. Older doctors who have worked in general practice for many years may well acquire these skills through long experience, but the new entrant should be aware that there is much to be learned and that patients will not be treated as well as they might be unless these skills are mastered.

Skills

The skills required are not difficult or unusual. They are based on a desire to manage a consultation, not by closing it down with closed questions, but by allowing the patient to say what he or she wants to say or should be saying, and to allow the patient to understand and cope with the problems that become apparent. The consultation itself then becomes therapeutic.

Every consultation except the most straightforward is a roller-coaster ride for both participants. The patient attends with an agenda; the doctor has none and must respond to what the patient presents as the problem. The doctor could be very apprehensive at the start of each consultation if experience did not indicate that most problems can easily be overcome. Acute pharyngitis can usually be dealt with by prescribing the appropriate antibiotics. It is the difficult consultation that makes the doctor's life miserable, but confidence in one's ability to manage any consultation leads to peace of mind and a reduction in the doctor's personal levels of stress.

Attitude

Doctors assess a patient from the moment that patient appears in the consulting room doorway, or so it is generally believed. If that is true, why should the patient not make similar judgements about the doctor? Is he or she likely to give them a sympathetic hearing? How much should the patient disclose?

The manner and attitude of the doctor dictate the style of the consultation, so the doctor's appearance is important. The way the doctor is seated, the facial expression, the demeanour, all are noted before the consultation begins or before a word is said.

The opening gambit

All doctors have a range of opening remarks that will encourage patients to unburden themselves. The remark could be anything as long as it is open. 'What can I do for you today?' might be a typical remark, and the result might be expected to be a straightforward presentation of the patient's problem. Often it is so, but not always. The patient may break down and weep for five minutes. The patient may counter with an equally open remark like, 'I don't know where to begin.' The patient may be angry: 'This is the third time I've been here with this problem', or the patient may simply say, 'Doctor, I feel awful.'

The attitude of the doctor should always be permissive until there is reason to be otherwise. If a patient cries, say, 'That's all right, people do cry here.' Reassuring remarks like 'Take your time' may help even though time is at a premium. Eventually, the patient will become composed and the consultation can continue.

The open question

The open question need not be a question at all. It could be 'Well?', or it could be 'Now then?', or even 'Uh huh?' It is an interjection with a question mark after it. It is an invitation to the patient to speak, or to say more. It is neutral and non-judgemental. It can be more specific, such as, 'What would you like me to do?' It does not express an opinion or a preference. It says to the patient, 'Over to you!' It allows the patient to say more without applying any pressure, and it is useful at the start of a consultation because it does not direct the consultation in any way. The patient is invited to lead the discussion.

The reflected question

If a question is asked by a patient, it is often advantageous to avoid a direct answer and instead seek that patient's own opinion. The question is reflected back to the patient. If the patient asks 'Do you think there is something serious wrong with me, Doctor?' it is often useful to ask, 'Well . . . what do you think?' It is sensible to be noncommittal, at least until the full facts are known and opinions formed, and it is always better if the patient can work out the solutions to his or her own problems. Patients believe what they hear themselves say. They do not always believe what doctors tell them.

Being noncommittal

Doctors are trained to be rapid decision-makers and making judgements certainly accelerates the consultation, but making decisions for the patient is not necessarily helpful. Some patients may wish to have early confident answers to their problems but making such judgements should be resisted by the doctor, who should never be afraid to say, 'I don't know.'

The use of silence

One way to force a patient to volunteer information is to allow silences to develop. Silence is a powerful tool, as almost everyone has an overwhelming urge to fill a silence, to say anything rather than let a silence hang in the air. A patient will often say more than he or she intended. Most new entrants to general practice know about the use of silence, but few actually use it routinely. It is worth trying; it is worth practising. If you think that a patient has more to tell you than is being admitted, use a silence. Just do not say anything; the patient will fill the space.

Unfortunately, there is an equal compulsion on the part of the doctor to fill an 'awkward' silence, so, if the patient leaves a silence it is wise to resist the urge to fill it.

Silence does not have to be intimidating. A patient may come to talk. A patient who was in the process of separating from his partner came to his doctor uninvited on a weekly basis and talked about his feelings and his problems, never really allowing the doctor time to say anything at all. After the separation, the man left the area and the practice, and later wrote to thank the doctor for all his help. The perplexed doctor had spent the weeks wondering why the patient kept attending, unaware that he was providing a service.

Direct questions

If the diagnosis is clear to the doctor, and if the consultation is going nowhere, it is allowable and often helpful to ask direct questions. If the doctor thinks the patient may be suffering from stress and wishes to clarify the situation, there is no harm in asking direct questions. There are some physical symptoms that almost all stressed or anxious patients experience. Asking about them can expedite the diagnosis and begin treatment. Examples of useful direct questions are:

- Do you wake up in the morning feeling rested?
- Do you feel that you have had a restoring night's sleep?
- Is your neck tight and sore in the morning?
- Is your jaw sore from clenching your teeth?
- Are your fists tight and do you have nail marks on the palms of your hands in the morning?

The previous discussion of the physiology of stress with particular reference to chronic hyperventilation explains why patients may be physically tense in the morning. A surprising number, almost all, will have the symptoms of nocturnal muscle tension. At some stage, a full physical examination is usually indicated, both to demonstrate the relevant physical signs and to reassure the patient that there is no physical abnormality. It is often possible to reveal painful tender neck muscles during this examination.

Using direct questions opens up the discussion about real physical symptoms and signs. This can have a liberating effect on the consultation, as the patient is enabled to participate in a dialogue with the doctor. Suddenly, there is common ground and the doctor seems to have an understanding of the condition and a prior knowledge of its effects. This does not always happen, but, when it does, it can be a turning point and the rest of the consultation may be much easier. It may be possible at this stage to explain the way these symptoms are caused in simple terms, to discuss muscle tension and to raise the subject of stress. Many GPs will know enough about the patient's circumstances to be able to anticipate the answers which will be given when enquiries are made about the possible causes of stress. In other patients, the cause will be related to work or other unknown family or marital circumstances. Airing a subject that has been previously denied can be of great benefit to the patient.

A list of common symptoms is given in Chapter 1. These can all be addressed and discussed if time permits, or the patient can be given another appointment and the symptoms discussed during a further consultation. If the patient continues to deny symptoms and also to deny the presence of stress, or if the doctor is in doubt about the diagnosis or wishes to confirm the diagnosis by eliminating the more obvious causes of the symptoms, further investigation is indicated. Thyroid function tests and a full blood count are a useful start. Initiating some investigations can buy time in a difficult situation, allowing the patient to return after a week. Relevant hospital investigations and even referral may be required if the diagnosis is not absolutely established. The diagnosis of stress is not necessarily one of exclusion; exhaustive investigation is not always required if a good history has indicated that the diagnosis is stress.

The co-operative patient

A patient who recognizes that the problem is stress and comes seeking help for that problem will be keen to co-operate in whatever treatment plan is devised and recommended. Long-term compliance is another matter, but there is scope for rational discussion, explanation and the giving of tapes or handouts. Such patients will be relieved that their problem has been recognized and diagnosed. If they have insight they will have anticipated the treatment methods that will be recommended. They will be prepared to look critically at their lifestyle and make whatever changes are appropriate and practical. The consultation is thus diagnostic and therapeutic in its own right, and the outcome will probably be successful.

The object of the consultation is to achieve an alteration in the patient's behaviour in subtle ways that will reduce stress. That does not necessarily mean seeking a divorce or changing a job, but it might mean taking more time to oneself, taking more exercise and certainly starting to do relaxation and breathing exercises. The informed and motivated patient will be happy to co-operate in these protocols.

The unco-operative patient

Some patients may find it difficult to fit into this model of the consultation or may see their illness in a completely different way. They may feel guilty or inadequate, or may simply fail to establish a rapport with the doctor. If physical symptoms predominate, they may assume that these are caused by a purely physical illness. Such patients may believe that they have a particular established illness, or they may invent an illness such as excessive catarrh irritating the stomach, or they may adopt an illness invented by someone else. Treating the wrong illness is never very rewarding and most doctors will resist an invitation to endorse an illness they do not believe the patient is experiencing.

There is great value in being noncommittal, as even the most apparently intransigent patients may come to terms with their problems if they are allowed time, often to the surprise of their doctors as well as to themselves. If the doctor cannot convince the patient that he or she has a problem with stress, or if the doctor cannot buy time, satisfactory treatment of the condition may not be possible.

The alternatives

If the patient is not knowledgeable about stress or about themselves, if they lack insight and awareness, or if they lack motivation, the doctor is in the situation of either giving up on the search for a satisfactory way of managing the patient or trying to convince that patient that the problem is stress-related and that managing the symptoms means managing the stress. As with every patient, appropriate investigations are indicated. Referral may also be necessary. Abdominal pain, chest tightness, headaches, dizziness, all of these worrying symptoms may require investigation, possibly to reassure the doctor as well as the patient. We are medical scientists after all, although the modern GP has an expanded role. If at the end of the day the patient still presents with the problem, how does one proceed?

There are several questions that have to be answered before a more determined effort is made to convince the patient of the nature of the problem and the requirement for treatment. Both the doctor and the patient must consider the following:

- Is there a problem?
- Is that problem significant?
- Would action be beneficial?
- Would the benefits of treatment outweigh the disadvantages?

Here we are entering the vernacular of counselling, which must exist somewhere near the peripheries of GP competence. We are talking about changing a patient's mind. Doctors do not usually adopt this role, allowing the patient to have control over decision-making, avoiding the risks of proselytizing. Doctors are, however, in the business of informing and guiding patients, but, if a patient does not have the concept of stress-related symptomatology, it is impossible for that patient to make a rational decision.

It is reasonable to ask a patient with a stress-related problem what he or she knows about stress and about what his or her view of stress might be. It would be reasonable to ask if it might be *worth* doing something about it, and if it would it be *desirable* to do something about it. Would it be reasonable to consider some small changes in lifestyle? Give the patient your view on the management of stress-related illness and then ask, 'Does any of this make any sense to you? Does it seem to apply to you?'

Another approach is to give the patient literature about stress and also information on relaxation exercises and lifestyle changes, and ask the patient to take that literature home and read it to see if it makes any sense. Is it appropriate? Is it helpful? Ask the patient to come back in a week and discuss it. If the patient does not wish to be treated for a stress-related condition, then that form of treatment is not practical. If the doctor and the patient can agree upon a way forward, then that agreement is an informal contract upon which future management will be based. It is upon agreement that all treatment is undertaken, whatever that treatment might be. Surgery, for example, is undertaken with the written agreement of the patient but no treatment of any sort is possible without the agreement of both parties.

The contract

Satisfactory treatment of any medical condition requires the establishment of a contract between the doctor and the patient, based upon a common understanding of the nature of the problem. If that understanding cannot be established, there can be no contract. The fact that there is no contract does not mean that the patient cannot be treated satisfactorily. Some form of treatment must be offered, as always, and it may be that the doctor will have to improvise and treat the patient symptomatically.

It is important that the physician does not conspire with the patient by endorsing an imaginary illness as these cannot be cured. If possible, the door should be left open for further discussion of the problem. A pejorative view of the patient's attitude is unhelpful. If at all possible, some kind of contract should be attempted, even if it means a 'fudge' or a compromise.

Treatment

In most cases, an amicable agreement regarding the nature of the patient's problem can be achieved with relative ease and the very fact that the matter can be discussed openly and fully is often the first part of the treatment. The patient may have made a tremendous effort to come to the surgery. For this reason, the ease with which a competent and committed doctor can describe and explain symptoms can be a great relief. The patient may have been isolated and besieged and for the first time there is now contact and discussion of the entire situation.

This initial moment of contact is of great importance, but it is not the end of the consultation and it is not treatment by itself. The patient will expect more. The doctor will have to provide more. What happens next depends upon the doctor's situation regarding the availability of time, expertise and resources. The patient should go away with some kind of help even if the doctor intends to refer him or her to a psychologist or other health care professional.

Further progress

Giving a patient insight into the nature of his or her condition is not the end of the matter; it is a start. Understanding will not reduce the severity of the symptoms, although it will reduce the worry and the isolation. More help is needed, either from the doctor or from other professionals. The choice of a management plan depends upon the severity of the condition being treated and the ability of the patient to co-operate. A GP's expertise is necessarily limited, as are time and facilities. Careful follow-up is essential but the investment of time is rewarding, and it is possible to treat patients by seeing them frequently for short periods.

In the short term, drug treatment for the acutely stressed patient has a place, but treatment will be considered later in more detail.

The bottom line

It would be wrong to advocate a prescriptive approach to stress management. There can be no mechanistic approach to the consultation. What is important is the attitude of the doctor, and the doctor's openness, desire to listen and willingness to help. Once this is understood by the patient, all things, or almost all things, are possible. The quality of the doctor's consultation technique depends upon that doctor's confidence that he or she can manage any consultation, no matter how difficult. That confidence comes from experience, practice and rehearsal, and the doctor's desire for professional extension.

Summary

- Consultation skills are vital in the management of stress.
- Consultation skills can be learned and practised.
- Patients differ in their presentation of stress.
- Patients have different attitudes to stress.
- The doctor and the patient have to agree the diagnosis.
- The doctor and the patient have to come to an understanding about treatment.
- Understanding stress is not enough.
- Patients may need further help from skilled professionals.

7

Somatic presentations of stress

The GP sees many patients complaining of conditions that are disturbing and, on occasion, disabling, but that appear to defy rational diagnosis and explanation. Such patients may be referred to a hospital specialist and exhaustively investigated before it is decided that they are not suffering from a condition that can be explained by traditional pathology. Hospital based specialists are as aware of this fact as GPs and regret that a substantial number of people seen in their outpatient departments do not appear to be suffering from a surgical, medical, cardiological, gynaecological or other category of illness.

Hospital specialists who are trained in one discipline are unable to advise on the treatment of these patients and they are returned to the care of their GPs, who then, as generalists, properly have the responsibility for managing them. This inappropriate referral and inability to manage a large group of patients presents a problem for the providers of health care, who see clinics being blocked by patients who cannot be treated. Specialists are frustrated by the fact that they see many patients who they cannot treat and who appear to be wasting valuable time. There is an understandable temptation to rationalize the situation by assuming that these patients do not suffer from the symptoms they complain of and that the symptoms are in some way imagined. It is easy to blame the patient for the illness.

The physiology

Patients rarely imagine or invent symptoms, although of course we all know that some do so and in the process acquire large folders of inconsequential hospital and general practice notes. In general, it is safe to assume that if a patient is complaining of a physical problem such as pain then that problem actually exists. It is on that basis that rational medicine is practised. A failure to diagnose and treat a problem is a failure on the part of the doctor and it does no service to the profession to attribute blame for such a failure to the patient. The fact is that the pathology is there and can be detected if the doctor looks for it.

The scale of this problem is immense. The number of patients presenting to a primary care physician with this type of symptomatology is put by some authorities as being as high as 50 per cent of the total. The reason why diagnosis and treatment appear to be unsuccessful is because the problem is physiological and is therefore a variation of the normal, rather than a distinct pathology; it is not a problem area addressed in medical schools or thus far taught adequately to doctors in training.

The nature of the physiological changes that occur in the stressed individual has already been presented and discussed in Chapter 5 and is briefly revised here. Blood gases, in particular carbon dioxide, are essential for homeostasis, but, at high levels of arousal, carbon dioxide becomes uncoupled from this function. With stress-induced hyperventilation, carbon dioxide is blown off, leading to a loss of carbonic acid and a resulting respiratory alkalosis. The body excretes alkali to compensate and maintain the normal pH. The alkaline buffering systems become depleted and lactic acid is thus unbuffered when it is produced in muscles as an endpoint in anaerobic respiration. There is an acidotic shift, which can lead to nocturnal hyperventilation as the body strives to lose more carbonic acid and secure homeostasis.

Hypocapnia has adrenergic effects, leading to a sympathetic/parasympathetic imbalance. Symptoms can result from this change, but hypocapnia has other effects. It produces hypersensitivity to stimuli so that an affected subject will experience photophobia and hyperacusis.

These physiological changes in turn produce a diuresis of magnesium, which is a calcium channel blocker, so that there is an increase in intracellular calcium ionization, creating an increase in the contractibility of hollow visci. This has profound effects.

The essential pathology that creates the symptoms in stressed patients is thus intracellular and fundamental.

Symptom generation

The stressed patient has three physiological problems: the results of sympathetic overactivity; a catabolic shift; and the sequelae of a magnesium diuresis. There is thus the possibility of the development of multiple symptoms, all of which have a plausible pathogenesis. None of the body's systems are isolated from the physiological changes that occur in the stressed patient, who feels ill and experiences specific symptoms that bring him or her to the doctor.

The patient may present in many ways and it may be of benefit to consider the possibilities system by system. Doctors are conditioned to consider presenting complaints systematically and medical specialties are more or less arbitrarily confined to such systems. The GP is by definition a generalist, who will see the relationship between particular symptoms and others that are less distressing, and relate these to the psychological history elicited from the patient. It is the GP who will make the diagnosis and institute treatment.

Symptomatology induced by hyperventilation

Doctors will be familiar with the sensations and symptoms of adrenergic origin and all medical students and just about everyone else knows about the 'flight or fight' reaction. Palpitations and other cardiac symptoms may be due to the beta actions of adrenalin. Most of the long-term symptomatology suffered by patients is due to the phenomenon of chronic hyperventilation referred to in the previous paragraphs, although not exclusively so. This hyperventilation is continuous and involuntary, and is usually unnoticed by the patient.

It is the symptoms created by hyperventilation that bring the patient to the doctor. The patient is usually unaware of the association between stress and the symptoms complained of, because they are apparently unrelated to immediate stress, and they are powerful and disturbing in their own right. The symptomatology will be considered system by system.

Musculoskeletal

Musculoskeletal symptoms can predominate and can be severe.

Diffuse or localized myalgia/arthralgia
Patients complain of neck stiffness and soreness, or of aching limbs. They suffer from tension headaches and wake in the morning with a sore neck, sore masseter muscles and nail marks in the palms of their hands from fist clenching during the night. They are prone to muscular aches and pains.

The most characteristic pain is in the neck and shoulders; if these areas are palpated they will be painful. This myalgia is a subacute tetany, the result of nocturnal hyperventilation. The patient wakes without having had restoring sleep and this effect is cumulative morning by morning until it becomes very intrusive. The nocturnal physiological shifts are secondary to the daytime problems, so, whilst it is difficult to do anything about the nocturnal problem, it can be treated by addressing the daytime problem. This can be explained to patients in a way that they will understand.

Tetany

Hyperventilation is associated with tetany; a degree of chronic tetany occurs in stressed patients. This may manifest itself as carpopedal spasm in extreme cases but it is more usually simple muscle pain and stiffness. The pain and muscular spasm can be severe and there can be a coarse tremor and muscle fasciculation. Acute tetany is more likely to occur in overtly stressful situations and is more common in young girls. It can be recurrent in children with school phobias but it can also occur in adults with social or work phobias.

Headache

Tension headaches caused by spasm in neck muscles are due to muscle irritability. The pain can be severe and protracted. On examination, the neck muscles will be tender and painful. The headaches can last for days; they can be very disturbing and refractory to analgesia. Patients frequently complain of headaches and children are not immune. Tension headaches are diagnosed on the history and examination but patients are not often receptive to the diagnosis, preferring to talk about their 'migraine' headaches. Patients do not believe that 'ordinary' headaches can be so severe or so long-lasting.

Patients can be told that tension headaches are caused by tension in the neck muscles and that the pain is muscular pain, which can be severe. Anyone who has had a muscle injury or muscle cramp in the calf will testify to that. This is an explanation that patients can accept.

Neurological

Neurological and psychological symptoms may coexist and can be confused. If a nonstressed volunteer hyperventilates neurological symptoms will occur. It can be assumed that neurological symptoms are real and that they do occur in stressed patients, although they are less precise and more difficult to describe than other physical symptoms. Hyperventilation can produce transient cerebral vasoconstriction, which could be assumed to be a mediator in many neurological sequelae.

Disturbance of consciousness

Subjects can feel unreal and detached and may describe these feelings. They may not describe them precisely or they may decline to describe them because they fear that they are odd symptoms and will not be taken seriously; they may assume that they are of psychological origin or indicate that they are going mad. Patients do have these fears and they can be allayed by the informed doctor.

Faintness

Patients may have feelings of faintness and, on rare occasions when other factors such as excessive heat are operating, they may actually faint. Fainting is a rare complication of stress but patients will often say that they feared that they were going to faint in a given situation. This is one way of interpreting their symptoms but there is a world of difference between feeling that one might faint and actually fainting. Patients may say that they feel faint even though their blood pressure has not dropped and they have not experienced syncope.

Dizziness and unsteadiness

Stressed patients may experience these phenomena, which they describe as dizziness or vertigo. They are upset by the sensation but not as distressed by it as a patient who has rotational vertigo. They do not have a central or a peripheral vertigo and will be unable to describe that symptom. The sensation of unsteadiness or dizziness is caused by an imbalance in the tension in the muscles of the neck. One side is tighter than the other and the patients feel that they are falling to that side. They feel unbalanced rather than dizzy.

Physical examination reveals unilateral muscle tenderness in the neck muscles posteriorly. Gentle pressure on these tender muscles may recreate the sensation of dizziness.

Impairment of concentration and memory

These patients are so 'self-conscious' in the literal sense because of the intrusive symptoms they experience, that they have problems concentrating on outside events and have poor recall of them. A stressed patient in a public place, or in a place where he or she may become flustered, will not remember very much about the experience. Fear of becoming flustered makes the reality of becoming flustered more likely. The more a patient tries to remember something, the more difficult it becomes; it is hard to concentrate and to remember.

Respiratory

Cough

Stressed patients may exhibit a cough or a chronic 'tickle'. This may be a habit cough but it may also be due to a degree of bronchoconstriction; it may possibly be due to hyperventilation. There are rarely any respiratory signs.

Shortness of breath: atypical asthma

Bronchoconstriction could also cause a true shortness of breath resembling asthma. This is not a symptom frequently seen and there are other explanations for a patient's respiratory symptoms.

Tightness of the chest

Patients often complain that they cannot get a full deep breath. They feel desperate and may throw open windows in order to get a breath, or go and stand in the garden in the middle of the night. This is a very frightening phenomenon, which brings the patient rapidly to the doctor. Clinical examination is usually normal and the peak flow rate is also normal. There may not be a history of asthma or bronchitis. The symptoms may be acute or chronic and there have been patients who have filled their bedrooms with fans and ionizers in the hope of warding off this symptom.

This sensation of tightness is due to spasm of the intercostal muscles, which will be tender on palpation. The patient's inability to get a breath is due to the constriction produced by spasm in these muscles. The chest is literally tight, or rather the chest wall is tight. Getting a full breath is difficult and the more the patient strives to breathe the more difficult it becomes.

Sighing respiration: excessive yawning

Abnormal respiration in the form of sighs and yawns is entirely typical of stressed patients. Most of the symptomatology is due to disordered respiration and on occasion this disordered respiration is very apparent. Improper breathing becomes a habit of which the patient may not be aware, although the patient's spouse may well be. Rapid respiration also occurs in stressed patients and this may be admitted on direct questioning by an observer. Controlling this type of breathing is an essential part of the treatment of stress and anxiety.

Cardiovascular

Many patients referred to cardiologists do not prove to have cardiac disease. Their symptoms may have other causes and this is a fact that many cardiologists understand very well. Disorders of cardiac rhythm are most common, but chest pain and transient hypertension also occur.

Palpitations

Stressed patients will sometimes complain of palpitations or skipped beats. This will possibly be a beta-andrenergic effect or it may be due to problems with muscle contractibility. It can be a particularly distressing and frightening symptom, which inevitably suggests heart disease to the patient. Palpitations can be long-lasting and may be present on examination.

Tachycardia
Tachycardia may be cardiac in origin or it may be due to peripheral vasodilatation, the former being due to beta-adrenergic effects and the latter to magnesium diuresis.

Atypical chest pain: precordial pain
This pain may be due to muscular contraction and irritability of the intercostal muscles, which may be tender on palpation. It may also be gastric in origin due to a reflux oesophagitis or to gastric hyperacidity. It is frequently due to dysfunction of the sternocostal joints, which may be secondary to intercostal muscle spasm. An individual sternocostal joint may be very tender on palpation and there may be chest pain on exertion.

Vasomotor instability
Stressed patients may flush or sweat, particularly in situations they find difficult or threatening. A rehearsal of the physiology of stress will explain this phenomenon.

Gastrointestinal

Atypical contractibility of hollow visci can produce significant effects on the gastrointestinal tract in stressed individuals. We have all had intestinal hurry in stressful situations. Animals are not immune and some horses will defecate immediately every time they are put into a horse box. Gastrointestinal symptoms are very common.

Oral dryness
Patients may suffer from a dry mouth due to salivary gland dysfunction. Again, this is a sensation that most of us will recognize, although we may not have considered the cause in the past.

Globus hystericus
This most dramatic symptom of stress is well known and well documented; it is due to a disorder of oesophageal peristalsis. Patients are aware of contracted oesophageal muscles, which they describe as a 'ball' in the gullet. They feel unable to swallow and keep trying to swallow to relieve the sensation. In doing so, they make the situation worse and may experience severe discomfort or even pain.

Dysphagia
In an extreme case of oesophageal dysfunction, the patient may not be able to swallow and may have to leave the table and vomit food retained in the oesophagus. The problem is worse if they are in company or

eating in a restaurant. It can be demonstrated radiologically as an oesophageal contraction, rather than a fixed constriction. Why hollow viscus dysfunction should be focused in one place, as it is in the oesophagus in this instance, is hard to explain, but it is a common form of stress-related illness.

Epigastric distress
Patients may suffer from epigastric discomfort or pain due to gastric bloating and gastric hyperacidity. There may be oesophageal reflux due to a disorder of peristalsis. There are many physiological reasons why a stressed patient might experience epigastric discomfort.

Aerophagia
Stressed patients swallow more air than nonstressed individuals. When this is associated with peristaltic dysfunction, belching and bloating can occur. Such patients may be excessively flatulent; this will make them uncomfortable, particularly when it occurs in company as it often does. Intestinal hurry does not help this situation.

Intestinal cramps
Peristaltic dysfunction will produce cramps, intestinal hurry or, on occasions, constipation; bowel habit is altered and cramps may result. One part of the bowel contracts against another and severe muscular pain results. Babies suffer from cramps because of the immature neurological control of their intestines. The control is lost in stressed patients and colic or abdominal pain may result.

Diarrhoea
In situations of severe stress, diarrhoea is common, as most people know. How many people have had diarrhoea before making a speech or going on stage? It is even more common in animals. The cause is an increase in peristalsis, which creates intestinal hurry and a liquid stool.

Genitourinary

Men and women experience different problems because of anatomical differences.

Frequency
Detrusor muscle instability may produce symptoms such as frequency, and disordered urethral function and neurological co-ordination. This produces difficulties in sphincter control, so that voiding becomes a problem. There may be frequency and urgency or retained urine in the urethra. Minor incontinence is possible.

Inco-ordination of the pelvic floor muscles can cause serious voiding problems in men, who will have difficulty in completely emptying the urethra, which results in pseudoprostatism.

Uterine cramps
Cramps associated with menstruation may be stress-related. Dysmenorrhoea is a condition associated with stress, which is, strangely, now seen less frequently. It has been suggested that this is due to modern society's more liberal and relaxed attitude to sexual matters, with a concomitant reduction in sexual stress. The uterus is a hollow viscus and thus prone to all the stress-related problems of such an organ.

Sexual dysfunction
Vaginismus and premature ejaculation are probably stress-related. Both can be caused by hollow viscus dysfunction, but the mechanisms are subtle. Orgasm and ejaculation require close muscular co-ordination, which is affected by stress.

General

Easy fatiguability
Generalized muscle tension and a lack of restoring sleep produces genuine fatigue, which can appear overpowering. Patients feel drained of energy and unable to cope. The condition may be termed 'chronic fatigue syndrome' although it has other names commonly used in the public domain. Fatigue is usually considered to be reversible tiredness, whilst downslope exhaustion is irreversible by normal methods. Patients experience nonrestoring sleep for the reasons already considered and they wake tired. It is very difficult for them to understand or come to terms with this phenomenon because they are not exerting themselves and they are getting a great deal of sleep; unfortunately it is the wrong sort of sleep. Patients feel tired because they *are* tired; they are 'tired all the time' (TATT). Some computers will store this notorious diagnosis in their disease registers. These patients will often be physically exhausted and very much in need of treatment.

Generalized weakness
Muscle tension is again the causative factor. Investigators have had difficulty in demonstrating an actual reduction in muscle power. This remains a subjective symptom that patients rationalize in various ways.

Frightening dreams
Dreams may be of psychological origin or they may be associated with nocturnal wakening due to compensatory hyperventilation.

Sleep disturbance

Sleep disturbance may occur for the same reasons. Nocturnal compensatory hyperventilation wakes the patient in the early morning. The essentially stress-related syndrome can therefore be confused with depression, which should not be diagnosed unless the patient has a depressed mood, because early morning wakening is not diagnostic.

In conclusion

The above symptoms may occur in combination and they can be associated with psychological problems that may complicate the diagnosis. It will take an astute doctor taking a careful history to make the diagnosis of stress. It is more important for the doctor to engage with the patient and concentrate on the individual problems than to concentrate on structuring the consultation correctly. A patient may need time and it is proper to leave a consultation open-ended if necessary, and see the patient on another occasion in order to establish the diagnosis and instigate treatment.

Some syndromes do not lend themselves easily to rational explanation. It would be most doctors' opinion that otitis externa and alopecia areata are stress-related disorders, as are pruritis ani and vasomotor rhinitis. Eczema and psoriasis are made worse by stress, as is asthma. Every doctor will have personal list of syndromes in which he or she feels stress may play a part. Stress has its effect not just at the physiological level but also at the level of the cellular immune system.

Stress and the immune system

Kiecolt-Glaser and Glaser (1991) considered the effect of stress upon the immune system in their book on psychoimmunology. It would appear that there is higher mortality in bereaved individuals than in nonbereaved controls. It is an interesting fact, for example, that a prospective study on men whose wives were dying of breast cancer showed a poorer proliferative response to mitogens following the death of their spouses, compared with blastogenesis data obtained prior to bereavement.

GPs may not be conversant with the minutiae of the immune system, but there is significance in the finding that, in the residents of Three Mile Island after the near nuclear disaster, there was a reduction in B lymphocytes, NK cells and T suppressor/cytotoxic lymphocytes. There was also a reduction in the number of neutrophils and in antibody titres to latent herpes virus. The relationship between stress and eruptions of herpes simplex lesions is well documented.

Very little is known about the pathophysiology of a fall below the mean level of immune competence with relation to susceptibility to conditions such as autoimmune disease, infection or malignancy. It is, however, of great interest that stress can produce such profound changes in the competence of an organism such as the human body. This knowledge would suggest that stress should be taken seriously as a pathogen.

Stress and longevity

There is some discussion about whether the effects of stress can be life-threatening, either in the short or the long term. Does stress produce permanent sequelae and does permanent stress reduce longevity? Do the physiological responses become pathological? The evidence seems to be conflicting, with much of the effort directed towards assessing personality type with relation to proneness to disease. Much depends on how one assesses personality. Reports linking specific disease-prone personalities with increased incidences of those diseases have been questioned.

Stress is more common in lower socioeconomic groups and thus in people who are more likely to drink and smoke. Myocardial infarction is more common in these circumstances, but there does not seem to be any direct association between stress and serious life-threatening illness. Patients can therefore be vigorously reassured.

Management

If the GP accepts that stress is important in the aetiology of many diseases, he or she is presented with a dilemma, namely, what should be done about it? Is stress to be ignored, or is to be assumed to be a contributor to many conditions and therefore to be treated on a regular basis? Should we treat a patient with otitis externa for stress? Should we treat a woman with dysmenorrhoea for stress? How do we treat irritable bowel syndrome? What is perhaps of more significance is that should society tackle stress in the workplace and the home as an important exercise in health promotion?

These are matters for public debate as well as for debate within the medical profession; yet there *is* no debate. Despite clear research evidence to the contrary, some doctors ignore the importance of stress and it is still not taught adequately in medical schools. For patients, treatment is a lottery depending upon the philosophy of the doctor who they consult and many will seek help from alternative practitioners, whose only contribution to their well-being may be to take their problems seriously and so reduce their levels of stress. Self-help groups fill some of the treatment gaps left by the established caring professions.

The treatment of the individual patient is always problematic, depending greatly upon the relationship and trust that is established between the doctor and that patient. Many patients would simply deny that there is a link between stress and the severe symptoms of their irritable bowel syndrome. Patient attitudes are important. When should the doctor treat a patient symptomatically, possibly giving sachets of dietary fibre to a patient with irritable bowel syndrome, and at what point should the doctor raise the question of stress, if at all? Will raising the subject actually help the patient? We cannot treat all our patients for stress, or can we, and should we? The practice of medicine is about judgement. In this generation of doctors, medicine is as much an art as it ever was. When and how to raise the subject of stress is always to do with judgement and patient expectation.

It is, however, a judgement that has to be made, and the doctor must use discretion. Failing to consider the possibility in an appropriate situation is to fail the patient. Failing to acquire the skills to treat it is to fail oneself.

Summary

- Stress alters the body's physiology.
- Stress produces physical symptoms.
- Symptoms have a rational explanation.
- Understanding stress physiology is the basis of treatment.

8

Psychological presentations to which stress can contribute

The human body is not designed to cope with prolonged stress. We have already discussed some of the physical outcomes of this. The fact that stress can also quickly develop into a number of more serious psychological disorders makes it a condition that requires to be recognized and dealt with both promptly and effectively.

It is probably fair to say that the development of most of these psychological disorders can occur over a much shorter period of time than is the case for physical disorders. Even a six-week wait for treatment can incur a disabling deterioration in the patient's condition. Here is an example of a stressed patient who has a panic attack one day, and has become severely agoraphobic within the week; this is not an uncommon scenario.

Case history 8.1

David is a self-employed painter and decorator, aged 44 and married with two teenage sons. Business has been slowly declining recently and he cannot see how he is going to maintain for much longer the standard of living to which his family has become accustomed. For weeks, this has been on his mind constantly, and he feels physically tense and tired a lot of the time. Three days ago, without any warning, he suddenly had a panic attack whilst at work, and was so terrified by it, that he went straight home, excusing himself by saying he suddenly felt sick. He actually thought he was going mad and was scared to tell his wife or anybody else. He spent two days in bed, explaining it away was a stomach upset. During these two days, a fear of going out of the house became apparent, so terrified was he of having another of these dreadful attacks. Today, he has tried to go back to work, but cannot even make it over the front door, because of shaking, palpitations and a feeling of acute fear and panic. His wife has called an ambulance, fearing he is having a heart attack.

Some level of anxiety is likely to accompany all stress; panic attacks are also surprisingly common. This can easily and quickly lead to one or more of the following conditions:

- Depression;
- Generalized anxiety disorder;
- Panic disorder;
- Phobias;
- Obsessions.

These outcomes are probably more likely when stress is chronic, but even a relatively short episode of stress can contribute to the development of one of these conditions. For many patients, this condition will remain even after the stress itself has disappeared. Phobias and obsessive compulsive disorders (OCD) are more common than once thought. Marks and Horder (1987) cite evidence that there are likely to be around 100 people with a disabling phobia or OCD in the average general practice population of 2000.

A problem currently receiving widespread media attention is post-traumatic stress disorder (PTSD). A particularly traumatic incident such as a rape, an accident or a disaster can cause some people to develop this very disabling condition. The patient does not necessarily have to have been personally involved in the incident itself. Merely witnessing a traumatic event or its aftermath can cause PTSD.

Many patients also become much more aware of their everyday bodily sensations, both normal and abnormal, as a result of an episode of stress, and this may account for many GP consultations dealing with patients who are worried about minor complaints such as vague aches, pains and sensations. Again, this behaviour can persist long after the stress that provoked it has been resolved, and can even develop into an illness phobia. Dwelling on these bodily sensations is usually the outcome of the patient's lack of understanding about the effects of stress on the body. It can also be caused by an increased awareness of their own mortality as a result of stress symptoms having been wrongly interpreted as life-threatening.

The long-term benefits to both GPs and patients of explaining in lay terms exactly what is causing the symptoms cannot be overstated for many stressed individuals. This idea was discussed in Chapter 4 and will be taken up again in Chapter 10. Armed with informed insight, they are far less likely to enter the vicious circle created by fear and ignorance of their symptoms, which can create long-term and more complex conditions. This is distressing for patients, and takes up a great deal of their doctors' time.

The risk of suicidal behaviour as a result of stress should also not be underestimated. Someone commits suicide every two hours in the UK; those particularly at risk appear to be young and old men. During the

1980s and 1990s, between three and four times as many men committed suicide as women. Unemployment, divorce, social isolation and family stress have been strongly implicated.

Bearing in mind that we have seen that anyone at all can be the blameless victim of stress, it is also true that anyone at all can fall prey to any of the distressing conditions already mentioned. Obsessional or phobic behaviour can happen to anyone, and can be seen in high-powered executives as well as in middle-aged homemakers. Patients are no more responsible for developing these symptoms than if they come to their GPs with tonsillitis or asthma.

It is hard to say what proportion of these psychological conditions is brought about by stress, as such figures are difficult to collate with there being such a complex aetiology. As doctors are aware, most of these conditions, with the exception of PTSD, can also occur in the absence of stress, perhaps brought about by childhood experience or a vulnerable constitution or personality. Experience suggests that a high proportion of the psychological conditions mentioned here do have a substantial stress component in their aetiologies. Even when no stress is evident at the time of consultation, the condition may have been triggered by an earlier episode of stress and is now sustained by fear, along with ignorance and misunderstanding about the effects of stress. It is also sustained and kept fresh by the daily repetition and revision of the aberrant behaviour. This is just like the old rote learning of arithmetic tables: repeating them every day, we soon became very good at them, and found them almost impossible to forget. Indeed, people who learn quickly are particularly prone to phobias and obsessions.

All of these conditions are of course best treated by a clinical psychologist or psychiatrist, who, in the case of panic disorder, phobias and obsessions, will most often use techniques such as progressive de-sensitization to treat them. This enables the patient gradually to relearn normal behaviour patterns. For phobias, this involves a process of approaching the feared situation a step at a time over a period of time. The agoraphobic will begin simply by standing in the doorway; once that is mastered through frequent practice, they will then progress to the end of the path, and so on. For OCD, the patient will gradually cut down on the compulsive piece of behaviour. Instead of checking the gas is off six times, they will practise checking only five times. In either case, relaxation and breathing exercises are used to reduce the feelings of anxiety provoked by these small steps towards everyday behaviour.

Let us consider just how common these psychological conditions are, and how easily they can creep up on the most ordinary of people as a result of stress. This may help to give a clearer picture of a range of patient behaviour, some of which may at first sight seem puzzling or even bizarre to the GP.

Anxiety and depression

These are probably the most common and easily understood outcomes of stress, particularly if the stress is chronic. It is easy to envisage how a stressful situation will cause anxiety, and, in the long term, how this can turn to clinical generalized anxiety, together with the hopelessness typical of depression.

In the course of a year, 12 million adults attending their GPs have mental health problems; of these, some 80 per cent suffer from anxiety and depressive states, most of which result directly from stress of some kind. One comprehensive review of the literature (Barlow, 1988) suggests that, 'Anxiety and depression are simply variable psychological expressions of a common biological vulnerability activated by stress.'

Rachel Jenkins of the Department of Health also asserted at a CBI conference in 1992 that the most common psychological illnesses are depression and anxiety, and that these are mostly caused by environmental stresses. This suggests that perhaps doctors should be even more alert to the likelihood of an underlying stress maintaining anxiety or depression. Successful identification and treatment of the stress could make a substantial contribution to alleviating these extremely common conditions and preventing more serious developments.

Panic disorder and phobias

Although an occasional panic attack brought about by stress can present little problem to some patients, for others these may become frequent and a source of great distress. This condition, now known as panic disorder, may even continue when the original stress has been resolved. As shown in Case history 8.1, panic attacks and anxiety can very quickly lead to the avoidance behaviour typical of a phobia. One review of the literature estimated a life-time prevalence of panic disorder of 2.3 per cent, and phobias of 13 per cent. In total, this means that, of those people known to us, more than one in seven will have a problem of this kind at some point in their lives.

The most common life-restricting phobias are agoraphobia and social phobia, not snakes or spiders as many people think. Contrary to popular belief, these phobias are in no way irrational. In most affected people, a fear of suffering a panic attack or other symptoms in public lies at its heart, not an unreasonable fear. People are not actually afraid of going out; instead, they fear the unpleasant symptoms or being embarrassed in public. For the patient, there is no logical explanation for the panic attack, so the initial, often terrifying, attack quickly becomes associated with where it happened, leading to a build-up of avoidance and further anxiety. The patient's unconscious conclusion is that, if no other explanation for the panic attack is forthcoming, it must have been something to do with where they were at the time. Alternatively, or over and above this, they decide that they must be going mad. This pattern of fear and mistaken beliefs again confirms the importance of explaining to the patient exactly what is happening to him or her.

Agoraphobia

Agoraphobia is an often underestimated and misunderstood condition, overwhelmingly affecting women rather than men, the reasons for which are not yet clearly understood. This may simply be because women are more likely to admit to it, or perhaps their often home-based lifestyle fosters its development. Often wrongly taken to be fear of open spaces, agoraphobia is in fact a fear of leaving the security of home, particularly if the person is required to go to crowded places or to wait in a queue of any kind. Again, it is the symptoms experienced when outside that are feared, not being outside *per se*. Unpleasant symptoms of stress experienced when out of the home become associated with being away from home, and a pattern of avoidance and increased fear can very easily and quickly spiral into a serious and life-restricting fear, as described in Case history 8.1. It is not uncommon for professional and business men or women to suffer from agoraphobia, yet still manage to function completely adequately as long as they have a car for travel. For those with agoraphobia, the car is often a substitute for the security of the home; they simply take it around with them wherever they go, like a security blanket.

Social phobia

Again, more commonly than is perhaps assumed, social phobia can develop in a similar way to agoraphobia. The main difference is probably that the situation avoided is that of having to 'perform' in some way in front of one or more people. Having to converse, dance, give a talk or demonstration, or eat or drink, may become a source of embarrassment or fear if visible symptoms of stress occur. Blushing, sweating, shaking, panicking, stammering, feeling off balance or light-headed can all be caused by stress, and all can encourage the avoidance of a range of social situations. The acid test of whether a social phobia is involved is whether the person can perform the required behaviour when alone, only succumbing to anxiety when other people are present.

Case history 8.2

Gary is a stressed young man who noticed that his hand was shaking a little one day a few weeks ago, when he was signing for something at the bank. He felt very embarrassed and avoided having to do so again. Then, a week or two later, his hand shook again when he was drinking with his friends, so now he avoids outings with his friends in case it happens again and they laugh at him. He is now so scared of his hand shaking, that his fear has made it happen more often, reinforcing the belief that it will happen. He feels that he is going to pieces, and now will not go out anywhere where his shaking hand may be seen by others. He has even begun to avoid eating with his family in case his hand shakes.

Such apparently illogical behaviour has a logical explanation. A similar pattern can explain why certain people find difficulty in meeting and talking to others, or fear speaking, acting or singing in public.

Even premature ejaculation and impotence in men has been included by some researchers under the banner of a social phobia, because of its obvious link to performance anxiety, in this case in the company of the sexual partner. After one failure to achieve or sustain an erection, perhaps as a result of stress, the man can be so distracted by performance anxiety that sexual arousal is reduced and the feared situation actually made more likely. A vicious circle again can build up very quickly. Vaginismus and lack of orgasm in women can sometimes be explained in a similar way.

Simple phobias

Simple phobias, such as fear of snakes, spiders, birds, dogs, cats and so on, are much less likely to be a result of stress. These are more likely to have been acquired through a fright or by copying someone else in childhood. There is also some evidence of humans being prepared genetically to fear potentially lethal creatures such as snakes and insects, and dangerous situations such as heights. Fainting at the sight of blood, injury or injections has also been explained as a primitive adaptive response to personal injury, which has the purpose of lowering blood pressure to minimize blood loss and the danger of shock.

Obsessive compulsive disorder

Many people, doctors included, have their own harmless and quite normal obsessions or compulsions. Many people simply have to put a pinch of salt over their shoulders after spilling it, will not walk on the lines of the pavement or under a ladder, must have ornaments or books displayed in a certain way, or find themselves checking twice that the gas is off or the door locked, even though they know they have just checked it. If these various needs are not met, such people suffer a pang of anxiety. This is the everyday behaviour on which OCD can gradually be built. Prevalence is difficult to estimate, as many never present for treatment through embarrassment or the constraints of the condition, but recent studies suggest it to be more common than previously thought, and may approach a rate of 2 per cent at any time. We are probably all familiar with well-known obsessives, such as the recluse Howard Hughes, but there is also likely to be one, perhaps less extreme, sufferer in an average street and many sufferers in the average GP practice. As already mentioned Marks and Horder (1987) cite evidence that there are likely to be around 100 people with a disabling phobia or OCD in the average general practice population of 2000.

Case history 8.3

Linda is 32 and works part-time in a sweet shop near her home to help make ends meet, as her husband has a very low-paid job. She also cares for her elderly grandmother, who suffers from senile dementia. Even though her grandmother goes for day care every day, Linda finds everything just too much, and has felt stressed for many months. Whilst her grandmother is at home with her, she has a habit of turning on the gas cooker and Linda is terrified of a fire or explosion as a result. One day, a few months ago, she checked that the cooker was off before leaving for work, but, as soon as she had locked the front door, she felt anxious in case the gas was still on even though she had just checked it. She thought she might as well make sure; it was better to be safe than sorry, so she returned to check. The next day she found herself doing the same thing, checking twice because she felt anxious if she did not make sure, and there was no harm in checking. This went on for a few weeks, until one day she found herself having to check three times in order to be convinced that the gas really was off, and to reduce her anxiety. Sometimes she would get half way to work, then have to come back to check. Now, after several months, she has to allow an extra 10 minutes to get ready for work, as she is unable to relax unless she checks four times that the gas is off before leaving. She knows this is stupid, but she just cannot help herself. The anxiety becomes so bad if she tries not to do it that she just cannot bear it. She is afraid to tell anyone in case they think she is going mad.

Obsessions are intrusive unwanted thoughts, ideas or impulses that recur repeatedly in a person's mind and are usually of a frightening or repulsive nature. Compulsions, sometimes known as rituals, are behaviours repeated to reduce the anxiety caused by the obsessive thought. Linda's obsessive thought was of the house blowing up due to a gas explosion, and her compulsion was to check that the gas was off. Likewise, if a patient has obsessive thoughts centred on a fear of dirt or germs, then they may compulsively wash and clean themselves and the house to reduce the anxiety caused by the thoughts. Other common obsessive thoughts include repetitive counting, blasphemous thoughts, or vivid images of harming or even killing a loved family member. The compulsions most commonly reported to Phobic Action, a UK self-help charity, include excessive hand-washing, house-cleaning, and the checking of water and gas taps and electric switches.

According to Barlow (1988) in his review of the literature, up to 80 per cent of OCD sufferers are also depressed, and, in a substantial number, a major depressive episode is present. It is hard to say whether the depression is a reaction to the disabling and life-restricting nature of OCD, or whether OCD is a manifestation of depression, rather than of anxiety.

Post-traumatic stress disorder

PTSD has come very much into the public eye in recent years, in the wake of recent air, sea, fire and other disasters. However, even going back to the First World War, the 200 000 'shell-shocked' troops were actually suffering from PTSD, and 20 000 of them ended their lives in psychiatric institutions.

Since PTSD is a condition that can follow an experience that is outwith the range of normal human experience, this may suggest to doctors that they will rarely see it. However, PTSD has been found to result not only from war and major disasters but also from such incidents as robbery, rape, sexual or physical abuse, violent crime, and serious accidents. Few doctors will have no patients experiencing such events, so people suffering to some degree from PTSD will inevitably appear in the surgery. It is also helpful to bear in mind that the degree of trauma experienced by an individual is not fixed by the seriousness of the event itself, but by how strongly the person reacts to it. There may even be a delay in the development of the disorder after the event, with symptoms not occurring for months or even years.

Although a full clinical assessment by a psychologist or a psychiatrist is required for a definitive diagnosis, it may be helpful for GPs to be aware of the nature of PTSD and how it might present to them. Here then is a thumbnail sketch.

In PTSD, patients will have experienced a traumatic event and have symptoms that have lasted longer than a month in each of these three areas:

- Re-experiencing the event through nightmares, flashbacks, hallucinations or intense reactions to similar events or anniversaries of the event;
- Avoidance of anything linked to the trauma, poor memory of it, or general numbing of emotions;
- Increased arousal, such as difficulty in falling or staying asleep, outbursts of anger, hypervigilance or excessive startle response.

PTSD can also lead to a depressive disorder, so, once again, the doctor should be alert to such a possibility when treating the depressed patient. Pathological grief has also been linked to PTSD, as the symptomology is remarkably similar.

This condition requires referral to a psychiatrist or a clinical psychologist. Treatment will involve a careful and systematic re-experiencing of the event, as soon as possible after its occurrence.

Summary

- Patients can become much more aware of bodily sensations as a result of an episode of stress.
- Patients can have increased death awareness as a result of an episode of stress.
- Stress can very quickly contribute to a range of more serious psychological conditions.
- Explaining the source of a patient's symptoms at onset can prevent deterioration.
- All of the conditions presented can happen to anyone.
- These conditions can follow on from stress:
  - Depression;
  - Anxiety;
  - Generalized anxiety disorder;
  - Panic disorder;
  - Phobias, particularly agoraphobia and social phobia;
  - Obsessive compulsive disorder.
- Post-traumatic stress syndrome can follow an experience outwith the normal range of human experience. It is not usually treated with stress management.

9

When to treat stress

All doctors will know that, if every complaint is labelled as being due to stress, the word will soon be out amongst patients and the doctor will no longer have a practice. 'Dr Bloggs blames everything on your nerves you know. I wouldn't go to him. If you want a good antibiotic go to Dr Smith. He won't bother you with a lot of daft questions.'

Alternatively, if you are a doctor and you achieve the reputation of being good for nervous troubles, a certain cohort of patients will seek you out. They are not all necessarily the patients you would wish to enrol on your personal list. A reputation for being good for nervous problems may be fostered by your partners, who see it as a way of getting rid of a group of difficult and time-consuming patients who may well also be incurable frequent attenders.

Such patients are difficult. Some may have personality disorders and be immune to treatment, but some will be sensible, adequate people crying out for help. Some may have become dependent patients because of one particular problem that has not previously been identified or treated. Some doctors do not know how to address these problems and some do not wish to know, but the well-rounded competent GP will want to be able to treat all patients as well as possible within the constraints of time, availability and resources.

General practice is just that: it is general. It is horses for courses. It is identifying a need or a problem and having the resources to treat it. A knowledge of stress management techniques is just such a resource which can be used by the doctor or built into the doctor's medical practice. It requires skill to manage stress and skill to know when such management is appropriate.

The general practice folio

If you have been in general practice, you will know something about it. If you have not had this rewarding experience, it will be a mystery to you. It is very hard to define general practice and explain what it is, and much harder to explain how it is done. Everyone has had some experience of general practice, either as a student or a hospital doctor on the receiving end of its referrals, or else as a patient. Like education, people think they know about it and understand it. Very few, and that includes some medical practitioners, do so. It is complex, skilled, tedious, very stressful in its own right, and sometimes very rewarding.

The intricacies of general practice derive from the variety and complexity of ordinary people, very few of whom have a good understanding of themselves. They frequently have no understanding of their own anatomy, physiology and psychology, and a very sketchy knowledge of medical or scientific techniques. The body of medical wisdom accrued over several millennia and passed on from generation to generation of physicians means nothing to them; why should it? They want, as they often say, something to make them better. They rarely welcome the suggestion that they will have to do something to make themselves better. Doctors advise patients to take more exercise, stop smoking and lose weight. How many do?

Making changes

People do not make changes in their lifestyles or thinking, because to do so is the most difficult thing in the world. It requires motivation, and it is not easy for a third party to provide exogenous motivation unless it is to a football team. Making changes is difficult, but it is not impossible. Insisting that people make changes alienates them and doing so is a well-known technique doctors use for getting rid of difficult patients: 'Come back and see me when you've lost three stone.' (Exit patient.)

Offering patients the facility, insight, knowledge and support that will enable them to address their own problems is different. That is an ability GPs should have. Just as important for the success of their practice, and for the satisfaction of their patients, is the knowledge of *when* it is appropriate to offer these skills. A GP may decide that one patient will never benefit from stress management techniques and so not offer them. That is a matter of judgement, but it is surprising just how often even the most unlikely patients pick up on the idea and benefit from it.

When to intervene

If successful treatment in primary care depends upon a contract between the patient and the doctor, it follows that at some stage in the consultation the doctor has to make the patient an offer. There has to be a bid, a suggested line of treatment, which the patient will consider, accept or reject. The offer may be a prescription for antibiotics based on a throat examination. The diagnosis is offered and agreed; the treatment is offered and agreed. That sounds easy, but most sore throats look lily-white and many offered diagnoses depend upon perceived patient expectations. Almost every diagnosis is problematic. A major factor in the offer a doctor makes is his or her understanding of what the patient expects or will accept; hence the complexity of general practice.

This understanding between the doctor and the patient may be built up over a period of time. The situation may be clarified by examination and investigation until the diagnosis is undisputed, but there are always treatment options to discuss and agree. Hospital doctors may lay down the law, but they should know that their patients go straight round to their local surgeries after their hospital consultations to ask their GPs just what they should do. There will be occasions when GPs will give patients permission to do exactly what they feel they want to do, even if it means ignoring specialist advice. Somewhere in this negotiating process is the possibility of an offer of stress management.

Introducing stress management

Advice and assistance with stress should be available to all, but it will not be welcomed by all. The suggestion that stress is a component of a patient's illness may be offensive to some because they feel that it suggests that they are 'neurotic' or in some way incompetent or inadequate. If the patient has not volunteered the information that stress is a factor, it is difficult for the doctor to know whether it is or not and even more difficult to know whether or not appropriate advice would be welcome. This is why stress management is different in general practice from the situation faced by volunteer groups, counsellors or psychologists, where the patient has elected to opt for stress management-based treatment. The GP is always in the front line, where the patient and the patient's attitudes are an unknown quantity.

If the doctor is confidently to raise the subject of stress management, it must be clear that stress is a factor in the illness and that stress management is important in the treatment. It must be clear that stress is contributing to the disease process from which the patient is suffering and that controlling that stress will be of real benefit. It is only after making that judgement that the doctor can decide whether the patient is likely to be receptive to the proposals about to be made and whether it is worth the investment of time and energy that embarking on this course will entail.

For the purposes of a discussion of these matters, it is convenient to divide the conditions caused or exacerbated by stress into three arbitrary groups: where stress is an obvious and admitted factor; where stress is accepted as being a contributory factor; and a group of illnesses to which stress may be a contributory factor.

Dealing with the obviously stressed patient

When there is consensus with a patient over any matter, management is greatly simplified. If a patient attends complaining of stress or of symptoms caused by stress the doctor's task is relatively simple. That patient is seeking help and will be delighted and possibly surprised if such help is immediately forthcoming. A meaningful history, a good explanation, reassurance, hand-outs of relaxation and breathing exercises, or the offer of referral, are gratefully received. The patient will be relieved and reassured.

Despite this consensus, it is important to choose words carefully. Jumping in with, 'Well, you're obviously very stressed' may produce an immediate and possibly involuntary denial. It is always better to let the patient do the talking. Even so, questions such as, 'What do you think may be the problem?' will almost inevitably produce the answer, 'I don't know doctor, that's why I came to see you.' The well-intentioned, 'You're not the only one with this problem, you know,' may provoke the angry reply, 'Well I bloody well feel as if I am.'

In every case it is better for the doctor to keep his or her powder dry. The best response could well be, 'There may be a way out of this, you know.' The patient then has to take the initiative and ask what that way might be, or express a desire to know more. The doctor is then in the less demanding situation of answering questions. The patient may ask, 'What can be done?' It is often better to explain that there are some conditions that cannot be treated by medication, which is the usual expectation of patients, and that the first step may be to discover just how the patient came to be in this condition. A dialogue then begins; it is this dialogue that will soon resolve the patient's problems.

When the *style* of the consultation has been established, when the dialogue has started and the patient is talking, treatment is under way and there will be an outcome that is more likely to be satisfactory than not. Often it is in the doctor's gift to give patients permission to feel the way they do. 'I feel such a fool,' is a common opening remark. 'Many people do feel the way you do,' may be a useful rejoinder, or the simple, 'That's all right.' The doctor may say, 'That's all right. I understand very well,' and then a silence will bring the rest of the story.

The doctor may have to encourage the patient and may have to communicate confidence to the patient with remarks like, 'I really do think that we can sort this out,' or even, 'I am absolutely certain, from past experience, that we can take this on and beat it.' It also depends on the doctor. It also depends on the patient. The important thing is to start a dialogue and keep it going in an atmosphere of support and understanding; that in itself is therapeutic and may even be all the treatment that is required. It may be enough to persuade the patient not only to take hand-out material home but to use it and practise it. That is no small achievement.

Dealing with the patient who has predominantly physical symptoms

With the possible exception of the patients mentioned above, the subject of stress management can be a minefield for the unwary or inexperienced doctor. The list of minor conditions substantially caused by stress is problematic, as no definitive list exists. Stress does not lend itself to lists and categorizing, but a possible list would include tension headaches, irritable bowel syndrome, dizziness, respiratory and cardiovascular symptoms, panic attacks and other conditions previously mentioned, including anxiety and depression. When does the doctor raise the subject of stress? Will treating the stress cure the patient?

One thing does seem to be clear. Treating the illness symptomatically without addressing the underlying cause is a waste of both the doctor's and the patient's time. If the doctor believes that stress is a feature of the illness then it is right to raise that subject unless the patient is obviously going to react adversely to the suggestion. Again, it is surprising just how many patients do have insight into their condition and possibly have a good understanding of it. They may need permission to be stressed or they may need an uncommitted third party with whom they can discuss their problems. Some will be convinced that they are seriously ill and will pursue their quest for a physical diagnosis as far as Harley Street.

It is not always necessary to confront the patient with a diagnosis of stress, certainly not during the first consultation. It may be possible to tell a patient with chronic back pain that relaxation and breathing exercises will help, particularly if everything else has failed. It is always better, if possible, to open the door on the diagnosis of stress and let some light in. The doctor may only be able to push that door open a matter of inches, but opening it at all is a start. The patient may surprise or amaze the doctor by casting the door open wide.

How does one raise the possibility of a stress element in a disease process when a patient is complaining of an itchy bottom? We might call it pruritis ani. How do you discuss stress with someone who has a discharging ear, or a runny nose, or tension headaches or abdominal cramps? Such patients want something to cure their symptoms; to the patient, that means a prescription. If the doctor feels that stress is an aetiological factor that is worth addressing, then it may be necessary to help the patient to come to share that diagnosis and become involved in that form of treatment.

Symptomatic treatment

Symptomatic treatment may be desirable and necessary in the first instance, and it may be the only form of treatment acceptable to the patient. Acute stress usually presents as stress, not as a physical syndrome. It is repeated or long-term stress that tends to become somaticized; the current consultation may be just an episode in a long-running disease process. A vasomotor rhinitis may have been treated as an allergy and the patient will have had steroid or vasoconstricting nasal sprays, neither of which will have done much to help. None the less, introducing the subject of stress earlier in the disease process would have been quite inappropriate; a process of treatment has had to have been followed before both the doctor and the patient have exhausted the options.

A once well-respected hospital physician used to advise patients with pruritis ani to sit on the edge of the bath and fan their buttocks with a copy of the *News of the World*. He was very specific about these instructions, but there is no evidence that his patients benefited from them. The climate of medical practice has changed since then; patients expect more and will accept more sophisticated forms of treatment. If steroid creams or suppositories do not cure the problem, and if an association with external stresses can be implied, the subject of stress management can be successfully raised. Stress management techniques are not as simple for the patient as treatment with the *News of the World*, but they have the advantage of actually working.

In conditions where a patient is experiencing pain, discomfort or any kind of physical symptom, it is appropriate to treat that symptom in the short term and hope to offer stress management in the longer term. It is also appropriate and possibly essential to investigate any physical symptom that might have a physical, non-stress-related cause. It is in the longer term, in the repeated presentation, or in the unsuccessful treatment, that stress management really becomes relevant. Only occasionally will a new patient with a new physical presentation request stress management.

When embarking on stress management techniques, it may not be necessary to mention the subject of stress at all. Sometimes important things are better left unsaid, providing they are mutually understood. The doctor might ask, 'Would you like to try some relaxation exercises?' The patient replies: 'Do you think they would help?' The doctor can counter with a well-chosen: 'Well . . .?' The door is open and the patient can embark upon stress-management techniques without having to discuss the problem. Whilst that is not ideal, it can lead on to a proper understanding between the doctor and the patient.

Stress and associated medical conditions

There are many grey areas in medicine. One of these is the degree to which stress contributes to illness in general and to some illnesses, mainly cardiovascular, in particular. In other words, does workplace stress produce hypertension? Does the stress of bereavement contribute to the incidence of coronary thrombosis? This leads on to the discussion of whether or not controlling stress would reduce the incidence of these diseases. This discussion could be far-reaching because it enters the area of disease prevention. If it is possible to treat an illness such as hypertension with relaxation exercises, would it not be possible to prevent it using relaxation exercises?

The relevance of stress in the aetiology of hypertension is problematic and depends to some extent upon one's personal philosophy. Nixon (1989) and Wheatley (1993) believe that stress is an aetiological factor in coronary artery disease and hypertension respectively, but there are many other contributory factors. Perhaps the unknown element is to what degree stress is a pathogen. Coronary artery disease is exceptionally high in Scotland, but does stress force the Scots to smoke more than their European compatriots, eat more greasy foods and take less exercise? If stress is in any way a contributory factor, should the community be practising stress reducing measures?

What should the doctor's attitude be to the patient with gastro-intestinal, cardiovascular or skin disease with regard to stress management? Should we be teaching all of these patients relaxation and breathing exercises? What about our anxious and depressed patients? The answer may be that the GP has an advantage over a more academic colleague. GPs have the reputation of being healers of the whole patient, thus anticipating the language of the alternative medicine lobby. GPs do not treat illnesses, they treat patients. The way a GP treats a patient is idiosyncratic and has to be so because it is based on individual judgement, which increasingly has to be seen to be an informed judgement.

It would be difficult, if not impossible, scientifically to select which hypertensive patients would benefit from stress management techniques, although such scientific methods do exist. There is a place for the pragmatist. If a farmer wishes to make a path from the byre to the stream, he does not employ an architect and a surveyor to draw plans and make calculations, he employs a man with a wheelbarrow to walk the route and make the easiest path. Sheep use the same system. If, in a GP's opinion, stress is deleteriously affecting a patient's general health, he or she should have the knowledge and ability to use stress management techniques to that patient's benefit.

What to offer

Stress management can comprise the offer of a cassette of relaxation exercises; it can be referral to a psychologist, or a community psychiatric nurse, or to one's own practice's stress management clinic. There is a lot of choice for the well-organized doctor, but what is appropriate? Every patient is an individual, so every treatment option is individual and tailored to that patient. This is particularly true of stress management, which is a personal matter. Everyone's perception of stress is different. Everyone's sense of individual vulnerability and exposure is different. Patients' needs are different and their requirement and acceptance of stress reducing measures is personal.

It is the doctor's expertise in assessing these criteria that is important. Expertise is acquired by experience, but experience will not be gained unless the doctor has the knowledge and courage to become involved in the patient's personal problems and motivations. If the doctor sees these factors as part of the patient's illness, then experience, expertise and success will follow.

How much should be offered? How far should a doctor pursue stress management treatment? That is for the doctor to decide in the light of his or her increasing experience. As always, it depends on the way the doctor interprets the signals sent out by the patient. These signals will be mitigated by the patient's knowledge of himself or herself, of his or her response to stress, and finally by his or her perception of the doctor, which is based on prior knowledge, the reputation of the doctor, and the progress of the consultation.

Summary

- Patients can be treated only with their consent.
- Patients will differ in their acceptance of stress as a diagnosis.
- The concept of stress must be introduced with care.
- The concept of stress as a pathogen may be introduced at any time in an illness.
- The greater the doctor's experience, the easier it will be to judge when patients will be accepting of the diagnosis of stress.

10

Treatment options

A GP should be able to identify a stressed patient and initiate some form of treatment. Doctors have always done so, but treatment should be appropriate and directed; this has not always been the case. Medical students have in the past not been exposed to the full remit of psychological medicine and have not seen psychological techniques as part of general medical services. Times change and patient expectations probably now demand that doctors should acquire this expertise. If the doctor is to intervene in a stress-related disorder, it is relevant to have an understanding of the dynamics of stress.

Figure 10.1 demonstrates a simplified model of the dynamics of stress and there are clearly several ways of intervening and several places in the spiral where intervention would be appropriate. It may be

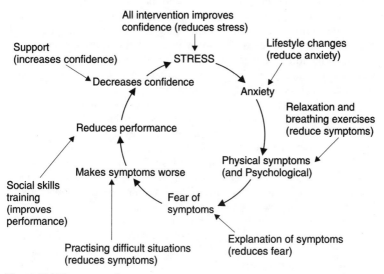

Figure 10.1 The stress cycle.

possible to remove the source of stress, but this is the least likely solution. It would be possible to intervene with drugs to reduce the symptoms of anxiety or to treat symptoms with specific appropriate drugs such as beta-blockers. Symptoms can be further reduced by educating the patient to control abnormal breathing and to relax tense muscles. It is further possible to teach patients about their stress, and how to manage the results of stress, so that they can cope more adequately and perform to their own levels of satisfaction.

In some of these areas, doctors might not feel confident in their abilities, but there is no reason why they should not take on some of the more basic forms of stress management to the advantage of their patients. The consultation, already discussed at length, is an important part of that treatment, but it is only a part.

Drug treatment

Drug treatment of stress has a bad reputation, largely due to the misuse of diazepam in the past, and possibly also due to the earlier use of barbiturates. Purists would argue that there is no place for drug treatment in the management of stress, but GPs live in the real world. If drugs are used sensibly (which must mean in the short term), they have a very definite place. It is the responsibility of the GP to ensure that drugs are used correctly and to withstand the pressure that can develop for repeat prescriptions, which is why diazepam was previously used in the longer term. Articles in women's magazines would almost suggest that these drugs were forced down patients' throats, whereas it was patient demand that created the problem of overprescribing. Drugs are part of a holding exercise, part of a broader picture of education and training, which is the real treatment of stress.

The benzodiazepine tranquillizers, mainly diazepam and oxazepam, are gamma-aminobutyric acid inhibitors, muscle relaxants acting centrally at cortical or subcortical level. They therefore reduce the symptoms so that patients rapidly feel better and so can cope more easily with their stress. They have physical as well as psychological effects. The main side effect is drowsiness, which is dose-related. In the much longer term, habituation may become a problem. Drowsiness is less in the longer-acting benzodiazepines such as diazepam, but it should be remembered that this drug will still be active 12 hours after it has been taken. Benzodiazepines, particularly benzodiazepine hypnotics, may have a depressive effect and so should be used with caution in patients who might already be depressed.

Buspirone is another anxiolytic drug; it is distinct from other anxiolytics, being a serotonin A1 agonist. It takes 10–14 days to act and so is not so popular with patients or with doctors. It reduces the symptoms of anxiety without psychomoter impairment and may have less potential for abuse than the benzodiazepines, although most doctors have a broad experience of benzodiazepines and can use them safely.

If depression is seen as a contributory factor, or even a potential problem, 5-hydroxytryptamine reuptake inhibitors offer effective treatment and may also have an anxiolytic function. They can make a patient agitated initially, but, unlike previous generations of antidepressants, they do work, and they are well liked by those patients who persist with them through the initial side effects.

Propanolol mitigates some of the effects of anxiety. A 10 mg dose or a long-acting preparation is useful, particularly in performance anxiety, and may have a place in the management of stress when performance is affected. They do not cross the blood–brain barrier and have no psychological action, but they do have a general inhibitory effect upon the peripheral arousal system.

Symptomatic treatment with drugs, such as analgesics, anti-spasmodics or gastric acid inhibitors, have a place in patients with specific symptoms if they make life easier for the patient. They are not a substitute for the treatment of the underlying disorder, the patient's stress, but they can help in the short term; any help is welcome.

Verbal advice

The doctor's main contribution to the management of stress is often to give the patient insight into his or her condition, and to offer reassurance and encouragement. This is by no means as easy as it seems. In essence, it is based on good consultation skills, which have already been discussed. Getting the patient talking about stress, understanding stress and doing something about stress is the basis of any treatment.

Advising about the patient's attitude to stress and any lifestyle changes that might help are also part of management. The most important practical help available to the patient is the use of relaxation and breathing exercises. These can be explained using the doctor's understanding of the physiology and how it affects the individual patient. If the patient knows that learning to breathe and relax will ease the presenting symptoms, then that patient will be motivated to try the exercises and persist with them.

It is important to encourage the patient to persist with these exercises; frequent review is desirable, if only to check that the patient is continuing to practise. It is here that nurses may have the advantage over GPs if they have a stress management clinic and time set aside to follow up patients. The patient presenting with stress will want some kind of treatment, and the most effective form of immediate treatment is the initiation of relaxation and breathing exercises.

Using printed material and audio cassettes

Research has shown that simply giving booklets to aid treatment of stress is effective, and is known as 'bibliotherapy'. The nature of such a booklet is given in detail in the Appendices. This deals with stress information, and with relaxation and breathing exercises, but it must be emphasized that it is used to reinforce the advice given by the doctor, not instead of it. The way this material is presented is important as it must be seen as a therapeutic tool. Patients will not read poorly produced or illegible material that does not excite their interest. Good material can easily be produced in any general practice, using the text provided in the Appendices and a word processor. It can be individualized for that practice. Appendix 1 gives details about the production of such material, and Appendixes 4 and 5 provide the text for written relaxation instructions and a comprehensive patient booklet.

This information reinforces what the doctor has said, as it can be referred to later, and it may give more detailed information that can be shared with a partner or a spouse and help him or her to understand the patient's problems, which may remove a frequent cause of difficulty. A small minority of patients will not have the intellectual ability to understand or use hand-outs, and their production takes up a receptionist's or a secretary's time, but the overall result is very satisfactory. Hand-outs move the doctor away from the simple reflex prescribing of drugs into another area of treatment, but the patient still goes away with something tangible from the consultation that seems to be important.

Relaxation exercises can also be provided on an audio cassette; this is relatively simple to produce (Appendices 2 and 3). An audio cassette is a much more practical proposition, as it is very difficult for a patient to read instructions whilst sitting in a relaxed position, particularly with the eyes closed. The practice can make a master tape (and some spares), which the patient is asked to copy at home, assuming that most patients will have this facility available.

The GP may wish to record someone else's voice on the tape, particularly for patients of the opposite sex, for reasons that should be obvious. A voice using the patient's own dialect, accent or language is obviously preferable.

Further treatment

It is one thing to have identified the patient who is stressed and to have initiated treatment, but what then? It is one thing to have found a relationship between stress and an illness that you have been struggling to treat for years, but what do you do now? The doctor may feel confident to proceed with treatment over the longer term and there is no reason why this should not happen. Further education may be available, or the doctor may have the confidence and the knowledge to continue, but there can be problems. Doctors are not psychologists. Their relationships with patients are different and multifactorial, and there are constraints of time.

Patient expectations play an important role in treatment provided by a doctor and patients may well not see doctors as people who treat stress. How often has a doctor heard the words, 'No offence, doctor, but I would like to see a psychiatrist. I need to see someone who will get to the bottom of this.' Patient expectations, based on Saturday afternoon television movies about Freud's Hollywood years, are almost never fulfilled and they may return dejected, but at least they have had their day in court, their opportunity to talk to a real psychiatrist. Likewise, patients raised on television medical soap operas do not expect their GPs to have any expertise beyond sexual prowess and an ability to diagnose leptospirosis in peripatetic ditch diggers. They do not expect their GPs to be able to manage stress; they may prefer someone else.

Referral

If a patient is stressed, or if the doctor has managed to demonstrate to the patient that stress is a factor contributing to the illness for which treatment is being given, that patient may wish to be referred for further treatment. The doctor may wish to refer the patient because of not having sufficient expertise or time, or because he or she wants the patient to have the best service available, which may well mean a referral outwith the practice.

Referral may be required because treatment is not being as successful as had been hoped, because the patient is becoming dependent, or because of a lack of co-operation by the patient or a lack of agreement about treatment methods or goals. It may be that the GP has identified stress and initially treated the patient very successfully, and in doing so has raised expectations that cannot be fulfilled.

The relationship between hospital- or community-based health care workers and the patient is limited by the fact that they are not available on a 'walk in' basis 365 days of the year. A psychologist may interview a patient and offer six sessions in total, and that will be the end of the treatment and the patient may not be seen again. The contract between a GP and a patient is open-ended and controlled by the patient on a demand basis. In practical terms, for most patients this is not a problem, but it can be. Occasionally, there is a good case, for reasons of self-preservation, for referring on patients who might be otherwise treatable in the practice.

Stress as an illness

In considering how far to take the treatment of a stressed patient, it is worth revisiting the condition in the light of earlier chapters. A case has been made for considering stress as a physical as well as a psychological illness, and of accepting a model of stress manifesting itself primarily as a physical illness that requires treatment. Stress can certainly be as disabling as any other physical condition and can create as much morbidity. It should be taken seriously by the physician and treated seriously, either by the doctor or by another professional. If that is to be the case, the doctor has to know not only something about stress but he or she must also know something about the other professionals who may be able to offer treatment.

These practitioners may work within the established health care provision, they may work in a university environment and be available for students, they may be provided by employers or trade unions, or they may be volunteers. They may, of course, be employed directly by the doctor's own medical practice. It is part of the remit of this book to encourage the establishment of such a service, which would be of immense benefit both to patients and to the practice.

A stress management clinic

Medical practices are now much more responsible for their own finances and they may, in some circumstances, have more choice in how they spend their money. It is possible to buy in psychological services, but it is equally possible to manage many stress-related problems within the existing practice establishment. With appropriate training and adequate resources, nurses and health visitors can treat minor to moderate stress; as confidence builds up, they can develop considerable competence. This is very different from simply asking practice nurses to chat to stressed patients in order to get them off the doctor's back.

Nurses work well to a protocol, and they relate to and empathize well with patients. With training and with proper back-up, practice nurses in particular, have a role in stress management, especially in the early stages of stress and with the less severely affected patients. Practice nurses will always be supervised by a GP, so there will be medical input and the patient is kept within the practice. There is no requirement to refer the patient to strangers or to a hospital, where there might be a perceived stigma, and where letters are permanently recorded in the patient's notes and may be used in insurance or employment reports.

Early treatment and a low-key approach to stress-related problems, together with ease of access, are important elements in a system of stress management. There is every scope for developing such a system in a general practice. Nurses are often keen to expand their roles and take on a challenge. General practice stress management clinics have been shown to work very well, as in the Stewarton Stresswise Project.

Community psychiatric nurses

Psychological services may differ from area to area and from country to country. Many GPs now have direct access to community psychiatric nurses (CPNs), who work in the community as a team in different parts of the psychology spectrum, from detoxification to stress management. They are available to see patients and to use the techniques outlined here in the management of stress. They will see and treat a patient and then return that patient to GP care.

CPNs are Registered Mental Nurses who have two years of ward experience before moving out into the community. They will have a BSc and commence work in the community as staff nurses to gain further experience. They tend to have special interests: in family therapy or behavioural therapy, for example, and they participate in an ongoing programme of in-service training in areas such as child abuse.

A high-quality community nursing team can be of great value in a primary care setting. The team will run group therapy sessions and bereavement self-help groups, and will deal with the problems of alcohol and drug abuse, which may be factors in a stress-related condition. Sometimes referral to the CPN service is exactly what the patient needs and wants. Occasionally, when stress is seen as a private and personal matter, the patient will wish to keep the problem within the confidence of the doctor. Even the most competent CPN service is then irrelevant.

The clinical psychologist

A few years ago, there were no clinical psychologist services available to GPs. In a short time, this service has grown and patients now have a knowledge of the role of clinical psychologists and a respect for their expertise. When a patient asks for a further opinion it is often a clinical psychologist whom the patient has in mind.

Clinical psychologists have a degree in psychology, and have undergone two or three years of postgraduate study, covering all of the clinical applications of psychology, including adult mental health, and physical and mental disability. Most psychologists will use a range of behavioural and cognitive techniques for stressed or anxious patients. In other words, they will make changes to the patient's behaviour by using methods such as relaxation and breathing exercises, and alter the patient's thinking style in the ways already described in Chapter 4. Patients suffering from phobias, panic disorder and obsessions are also treated in the ways described in Chapter 8.

It must again be emphasized that, after a number of sessions with a clinical psychologist, the patient is returned to the care of the GP. It is useful if the GP has a knowledge of the techniques used by a psychologist and can reinforce what has been done.

The counselling psychologist

The employment of counselling psychologists is a very recent development, which may not yet be available in many areas. In general terms, such counsellors come from a broad-based background with a first degree in psychology and several years of postgraduate training or experience in one or more perspectives of counselling.

Counsellors

Anyone can call themselves a counsellor at the present time, so great care must be taken when referring patients or taking on a counsellor in the practice. Most counselling tends to involve talking through problems in the here and now, in a supportive and empathic relationship. Having said that, there is a range of perspectives within counselling, with widely differing views on what counselling should comprise. Those who are suitably qualified can come from a range of backgrounds, such as nursing, social work, voluntary work, and so on.

No matter what the counselling style, or whether counselling is practised within or outwith general practice, the crucial aspect for the GP to be clear about is what exactly is being offered to the stressed patient. If the majority of the standard stress management techniques, as described in Chapter 4, are not included, which is likely to be the case, then the counselling on offer is likely to be inadequate for most patients. In general, counselling is not advice-giving. Stressed patients need clear practical advice, and lots of it. Counselling, therefore, must not be seen as a panacea for patients whose problems are not purely physical in origin, and particularly not for stress.

What *can* counselling offer the stressed patient? For a substantial minority of patients, counselling may have a useful complementary role to add to stress management advice by:

- Giving essential sustainment to those patients who lack social support, whilst helping them to develop their own support networks;
- Helping patients to clarify the source of their stress, and whether they can do anything to reduce or remove it;
- When the patient's personality, thinking style, or past history lays him or her open to stress, offering the opportunity to explore this further if required, and choose appropriate action (as discussed in Chapter 4).

It goes without saying that referral to private counsellors, other than those whose methods are clearly explained and acceptable, and whose qualifications are accredited by a recognized authority, is to be avoided.

Voluntary groups and self-help

In many areas of the UK, patients will have access to advice about managing stress through local self-help groups or advice centres. A list of central contact addresses for relevant organizations is given in Appendix 6. Doctors might consider providing this contact information to patients, or including an appropriate selection of contact details in their patient leaflet, if they decide to produce one.

There is a wide range of self-help organizations, most of which provide sound advice together with important support. Such provision does tend to be patchy throughout the country. As usual, it is advisable to check that what is being provided by such organizations is sound before encouraging patients to take up their services.

Some patients will not even need the support of such groups, but, once aware of their problem, they will be able to help themselves simply by gaining access to appropriate books and tapes on managing stress, either by buying them or borrowing them from the local library. A list of useful resources of this kind is included in Appendix 7; it also forms part of the text for a patient booklet, as given in Appendix 5.

Local adult education courses in stress management

Again, provision is patchy, but many patients will also have access to well-organized stress management courses or relaxation groups run by adult or community education services or their equivalent, or by health promotion or other statutory bodies. Many universities and colleges also now engage in outreach work in local communities, which may include courses in stress management and assertiveness. Advice centres, community projects specifically aimed at improving general or mental health, and women's centres are all likely to run courses. These are particularly common in areas of deprivation, where many courses are free. Most others carry a small fee per session, possibly with reductions for those on low incomes.

Here also, it is useful to check out exactly what is being provided by a course, as this can vary substantially. Information about courses is usually easy to find, as they advertise widely and may well circulate leaflets among local general practices. The main drawback with all of these courses is that they tend to be restricted to certain times of the year, often during traditional term times, whereas patients, of course, do not conveniently present themselves in the surgery according to a timetable.

Alternative therapists

All GPs know about the proliferation of alternative therapists, and all will have their own views on the subject. A growing number of GPs themselves practise an alternative therapy, such as hypnosis, as an effective adjunct to their other skills. There is no time and no need to go into detailed discussion on how each alternative therapy may or may not be useful for stress. Suffice it to say that most, if not all, of these therapies are not adequate in themselves to deal effectively with stress. Independent alternative therapists frequently claim to offer the miracle cure for stress; none provide it, unless they include the majority of the stress management techniques detailed in Chapter 5.

What appropriately qualified and accredited therapists, whether independent or not, *can* do is to contribute to the patient's overall management of stress. For the patient who lacks social support, they can be the ones who provide it. Counselling, already discussed, is especially valuable for this, and also for allowing the patient to explore issues surrounding the cause of their stress. Alternative therapy can also be the source of a regular enjoyable break, especially if some form of relaxation is involved. Aromatherapy and reflexology are becoming increasingly popular with patients for this purpose.

All of this can be an effective and important contribution to managing stress for many patients. Just having someone who will give them space and regular one-to-one attention, no matter what the alternative therapy used, is likely to reduce both existing stress and the vulnerability to future stress.

Occupational health services

Satisfactory occupational health services are rare. Where they do exist, they tend to represent the interests of employers. In such places as the Civil Service there can be helpful doctors who will negotiate with managers on behalf of patients who are stressed. It is sometimes worth asking if there is an available occupational health service, particularly if there is occupational stress. Some white collar workers will be in private occupational health schemes and have quick access to private psychologists, which can be useful.

Universities often have medical centres with resident psychologists, but students may be unaware of this fact and go home for treatment. Again, university doctors are well placed to discuss student health problems with tutors, which can be of great importance for a stressed student. Advising a student to contact a university health centre can therefore be helpful.

The doctor

At the end of the day, it is the GP who has to continue the relationship with the patient. For other therapists, treatment is an episode, and the patient one of many. For the family doctor, that patient will return, perhaps in pregnancy, perhaps in a terminal illness, or in a further episode of stress occurring spontaneously, or possibly triggered by bereavement or divorce. As in so many situations, in the long term it is the GP who picks up the pieces and helps the patient to carry on.

Every GP does manage these situations because there is no choice, because the patient cannot be referred every time, because it just is not possible to refer patients with minor stress. Other professionals have taught patients how to manage stress themselves, and many believe that they will be self-sufficient, but GPs know different. Patients *do* come back, looking for support, if nothing more. A GP must know something about stress management and something about the techniques used by other professionals.

It is important that the GP should avoid creating a dependent patient or a frequent attender, and so must encourage the patient to seek support from family, friends, church or volunteer groups. Stress is endemic in our society and educating patients to manage its long-term effects is important. If a patient keeps attending over years, wishing to engage the doctor in more and more of his or her ongoing stress-creating problems within the family or the workplace, it is reasonable for the doctor to explain that the remedy has been explained, that the treatment is available, and that the patient has again to address those problems that are causing the distress.

Ultimately, it is not part of a doctor's job to listen to a patient's endlessly rehearsed problems. The informed doctor offers a method of treatment and it is up to the patient to use that treatment. It is the patient's responsibility to deal with these problems, and, if he or she does not choose to comply with the treatment offered, it is that person who has missed the opportunity and who must live with the consequences.

Summary

- The GP initiates treatment.
- The consultation is the cornerstone of treatment.
- It is permissable to use drugs in the short term.
- Stress management clinics can be established in general practice.
- Patients can be referred.
- Long-term management tends to be the responsibility of the GP.

11

General practitioner stress

General practice is a stressful occupation. The results of such stress are apparent to all in terms of illness, broken marriages, alcoholism and suicide, but, for most GPs, the daily stress of their occupation manifests itself in less dramatic ways. It would be unrealistic to discuss the management of stress in others without recognizing, confronting and managing the stress in ourselves. This is something at which GPs are particularly bad. There is an inherited tradition of the macho GP, the doctor who can manage any situation and deal with it, who can work by night and day and deal with trauma, depression, bereavement and anger in others without any personal cost. That tradition is slowly changing.

Stresses in general practice

The causes of stress in general practice are more subtle than many doctors believe. Hospital medicine is stressful and, for a surgeon carrying out life-saving surgery or an obstetrician charged with the responsibility of always delivering a healthy child, general practice may seem relatively low-key. Indeed, the acute stresses created by emergency situations are relatively infrequent and are becoming less so with the development of paramedical services. Many doctors would now agree that a team of paramedics with modern equipment deals better with most medical emergencies than a single-handed doctor. Cardiopulmonary resuscitation is fine in theory, but exhausting in practice, and keeping skills up to date is a major problem better dealt with by the ambulance service.

Doctors do attend emergencies and this is usually a traumatic experience. The emergency may be in a public place. The doctor is perhaps known to the onlookers and to the family of the patient; a great deal is expected and often not delivered because there is nothing to be done. The difference between the GP and a paramedic exemplifies the problems that GPs face compared with other doctors or health professionals.

The GP is the 'family doctor'. After the emergency, the doctor has to look after the family and follow up the situation, whilst the emergency services return to their duties. What is possibly worse than this, and is in a bizarre way more stressing is that the GP will have lost part of an already full day. Whilst that may be of no significance to the participants in the emergency, it is of relevance to the patients sitting irritably in the waiting room or waiting for house calls. The fact that someone has just died is of no interest to them at all, and properly so. There is no benefit to the doctor or the patient if one situation is carried over into the next.

It is with these administrative and logistical problems that stress develops. It may be the requirement to deal with the same intensity with a terminal event as with the sore throat from which a cheeky, impossible child is supposed to be suffering. A doctor is as good as his or her last consultation. The parent of the child with the third reported sore throat in a month will expect satisfactory treatment, even if the throat appears aggressively normal to the doctor. Something will always have to be done. Parents and patients make no allowances for a doctor's problems and literally do not want to know. Patient expectation is a source of stress.

There is an abundance of literature on industrial and business stress, some of which is relevant to general practice. There is now a counselling industry, and counsellors who deal with stress are advised how to avoid stress in themselves. General practice is unusual in that there is no occupational health service and doctors have to manage in a tradition of self-sufficiency which is wholly inappropriate to the nature of their occupation, charged as it is with stress-inducing problems. It is worth considering these problems in detail.

Sources of stress: organizational

Lack of structure in the working day

General practice is a demand-led service. It is very difficult to plan anything in advance. A surgery may be straightforward or it may be long and difficult and full of interruptions. There may be 10 house calls or there may be none. A partner may be away at a meeting or at court; there may be a sudden death or a patient to be committed under the Mental Health Act. Unpredictability may be an advantage in some ways, but, when there is work to be done, uncertainty and an inability to plan can be stressful. If a day has been planned in advance and has certain demands upon time, constant diversions that make adherence to the timetable impossible can be very frustrating.

Time management

Coupled with the lack of structure in the day is the built-in inability to manage time. In terms of a simple surgery, there would be no problem if every patient required exactly 10 minutes of the doctor's time, but some patients take less, and some take more. Some patients are simply long-winded and like to talk or refuse to come to the point. Others will be depressed or have emotional problems and will require time and attention. A five-minute appointment can last for half an hour. Often the patient who complains about a long wait in the waiting room is the one who takes 10 minutes to discuss the weather before broaching the subject of the reason for the visit.

Doctors are very aware that patients are waiting. The knowledge that some patients have been waiting for half an hour is very destructive to the consultation process and many doctors become quite agitated. Ten minutes seems to be a watershed. Patients waiting less than 10 minutes do not constitute a problem for the GP. Longer than that, and the GP tends to become stressed. There have been efforts to solve this problem by asking patients to estimate how long their consultation will take, or by asking patients to book a double appointment if they have a lot to discuss. Patients are poor at time prediction and no one can know when a simple problem will lead on to a complex and problematic consultation lasting a long time.

Interruptions

Many people can make claims on a doctor's time. One of the primary functions of a doctor is decision-making; decisions may be required by receptionists, patients or nurses at any time. Many people feel that their requirement for answers takes precedence over other matters and there is an urge to interrupt the doctor, thus also intruding on his or her train of thought. Constant interruptions lead to increasing stress, frustration and anger.

Doctors are, of course, often interrupted for significant reasons, such as the occurrence of an emergency or the need to be consulted by a law officer or a medical specialist.

Administration

The vast increase in administration that occurred after the 1990 Contract was introduced in the UK has become a major cause of stress for doctors. Most do not like administration; some may be good at it, others are not, and it can accumulate. Administration of fundholding and other changes can take up a great deal of time, which might be better invested in patient care. Many of these imposed changes seemed meaningless; in particular, the necessity for recording health promotion data was seen as being a total waste of time. Being forced to do work that is perceived as being useless erodes morale and creates stress. A pile of uncompleted forms lurking on a desk somewhere can be very stressful.

Sources of stress: patient attitudes

If every patient was pleasant and empathetic, the life of a GP would be idyllic, but this is not the case. Every member of our society has the right to have a doctor and they nearly all exercise that right, so patients come in all shapes and sizes and are of all types. Some are pleasant and some are not. The doctor will actively dislike some patients. The patient's attitudes to life may be the antithesis of the doctor's or the patient may be filthy, aggressive, suspicious, arrogant or violent. The doctor will have to adopt a neutral position and attempt to assist the patient, despite his or her own prejudice. This is perfectly possible, but it is very stressful because the doctor must keep this prejudice hidden from the patient. This can be a difficult or demeaning task.

Patients may also be over-friendly and assume a relationship that does not truly exist. The doctor may simply detest the patient and hope that this dislike does not show. How many of these gratuitously friendly patients know that their doctor actively dislikes them? Their news-agents, bank managers and binmen may take the same attitude, but the relationship with the doctor is more intense and can often be intimate. It is therefore more demanding and stressful for the doctor than for other individuals.

Another demanding encounter is with the manipulative patient, the patient who has a different agenda for some personal reason, or perhaps just from habit, and wishes to involve the doctor in a concept of life or medical care that has little relationship to the actuality. That patient's agenda may be the desire to extract money from the State or the insurance industry, but it is just as likely to be to gratify some personal desire. Often, it is a wish to receive recognition for an illness from which the patient does not suffer, or it may be the need for medical recognition of the fact that a partner is unkind or uncaring, or that an employer is unjust. The doctor may decide to agree to this requirement, or resist the manipulation. In either case, the doctor feels uncomfortable and stressed.

Difficult patients come in all sorts, from the bad to the mad to the plain irritating. They create difficult consultations over which the doctor has little control and which are thus frustrating and stressful.

The incompetent patient

A list of difficult patients would not be complete without mention of the incompetent patient with whom communication is difficult. Such patients may be frequent attenders with unresolvable problems, who have turned to the doctor as a source of support. They cannot be helped and they are dependent. They may be cheerful or they may be sad. They are time consuming and contact with them can be frustrating and often stressful for the doctor.

The ill patient

No doctor minds seeing an ill patient; doing so can be fulfilling and satisfying. Seeing three of four depressed patients in one surgery can be depressing in itself; this is something GPs often have to do. The same may be true for very ill patients. Doctors have little protection from the trauma these repeated encounters can bring.

There are ways of protecting oneself from such stress, but doctors will often deliberately engage with ill patients in order to help them. In managing a terminally ill patient, a doctor will often deliberately form a relationship with the patient and his or her family by attending frequently so that such constant care becomes part of the patient's life and is as such unremarkable. The doctor 'looks in' every day, sometimes just to talk about the weather, so that, when big decisions about management have to be made, the doctor is in a position to make those decisions. When a patient dies, it can be distressing. This is a frequent and repeated occurrence for a GP.

It is possible to take a detached and professional stance and one does, but it is not possible to isolate oneself completely from the suffering of the patient and the patient's family. Doctors would not wish it any other way. The doctor will create an environment where the patient may ask difficult questions and seek difficult answers; it is not unknown for a doctor to leave a patient's bedside in some distress.

Modern theories of medicine suggest that a doctor should be able to share this emotion with a patient and be prepared to cry if necessary. In some cultures, this approach might be acceptable, but it is more likely that a patient will be happier with the more conventional model of the doctor, that of a caring professional. What is more difficult is the requirement to readjust emotionally almost instantaneously and to greet the next patient as if he or she was the first of the day.

If a doctor hears, overhears or is advised of criticism, it is not usually about the quality of terminal care, it is about an inability to cure a sore throat, a sore back or excessive catarrh, or the failure of some minor administrative procedure outwith the doctor's control. The patient's perception of a doctor's role is a personal perception mitigated by individual expectations. The doctor must therefore always remember to smile and produce the appropriate responses however bizarre the patient may appear. It's what the patient thinks that matters.

Reacting to patients

The problem of engaging with 20 patients in quick succession, responding appropriately to their demands and providing them with individual and reassuring treatment, is not easy. If four of them are depressed, it is more difficult. If a few are dependent, or if seven in a row (it has happened) are complaining of low back pain, then the morning can become impossible and certainly stressful. If the doctor is in good form, it is manageable; if the doctor is tired or preoccupied with personal problems, it is impossible or at best very stressful.

It is the constant engaging and disengaging with patients that takes its toll. It is hard not to feel 'two-faced' when one responds almost instinctively and differently to the appearance of the next patient in the doorway of the consulting room, and produces appropriate responses for that individual patient. Yet, if the doctor is to do the job, he or she has to take short cuts. That means adapting to the individual patient's vernacular and expectations. There is not time to allow the patient to develop an understanding and an acceptance of the doctor's position. The doctor tends to adapt to the patient rather than vice versa, which can be difficult and stressful.

Boredom

Some problems will not be admitted readily by some doctors, even to themselves or amongst colleagues. Medicine is like many other occupations: hours of boredom followed by extreme excitement. Both can be stressful and the transition always is. It must be true that many patients would not qualify as personal friends, neither would their complaints be particularly interesting. Patients always imagine that their notes are full of interesting observations, but there is nothing less interesting than a pile of patient records. No one, and no one's illness or complaint is as interesting as that person thinks it is.

When patients attend following a road traffic accident and are asked what the problem is, they will always launch into a detailed explanation of the events of the accident. Sometimes they have sustained minor injury and sometimes no injury at all. It is the nature of the accident that enthrals the patient, but not the doctor, who has heard it all before and who may be running very late.

Patients do not understand that a doctor has experience of illness, that virtually no situation is new, and that he or she has almost certainly heard it all before. Thus, patients like to describe their coughs in precise and graphic detail. Listening to such a description may be part of the treatment, but it is boring, particularly if the doctor has heard it five times already that morning. The intimate nature of the doctor/patient relationship, and the necessity to allow the patient free expression, can be very demanding on the doctor.

Complaints

Patients have been rightly encouraged to complain about the activities and failures of their doctors and some avail themselves of the opportunity to so do. Doctors know that the complaining patient is not the patient who *should* complain (the one about whose treatment the doctor is embarrassed), it is the patient for whom everything possible has been done and who seems wilfully to misunderstand the intentions and expectations of the medical practitioner. Every individual on earth makes mistakes and doctors are no exception. The only way not to make mistakes, or errors of judgement as they could be called, is not to practise at all. Patients are on the whole very understanding and forgiving of errors of judgement made in good faith. Occasionally, patients or their relatives do make formal complaints. Righteous indignation is a powerful human emotion and a wronged patient will pursue a doctor to the ends of the earth.

The fear of a complaint, or the expectation of a pending complaints hearing, has become a major source of stress in modern general practice. There are documented accounts of tragic suicides attributable at least in part to pending legal or quasi-legal proceedings.

Drug abusers

In recent years, drug abusers have become a problem in general practice. Most doctors are now plagued by addicts who hope to beg a prescription for a few tablets from the unwary or sympathetic doctor. Addicts are often popularly characterized as innocent youngsters who have been led astray, whereas they tend more often to be manipulative psychopaths who use drug addiction as a way of achieving power or profit. They are persistent, unscrupulous and potentially dangerous. Their presence in the streets and in the consulting room is a source of stress that doctors could well do without. It is not uncommon now for GPs to attend courses on self-defence. It is unfortunate that this should be seen as being necessary and it is an obvious source of stress. The doctor going to meet a patient at night, at a place and a time of the patient's choosing, and carrying a bag containing ampoules of diamorphine and pethidine, is a bizarre concept incompatible with the times in which we live.

Night work

Working at night in the conventional GP mode brings the dangers of assault, but there are more mundane problems. Being 'on call' means working; being on call at night means not sleeping, or certainly not getting a restoring night's sleep. Working after a full day's general practice is exhausting, and working more hours after a full day's work and a night on call compounds the problem; fatigue becomes constitutional and chronic.

The fear of assault at night is a further aggravation, but worse still is the casual way in which GPs in the UK are now called out of hours. No matter is too trivial for the patient to demand a night visit. The more trivial it is, the more aggravated the doctor feels. No doctor sleeps well after being called out of bed to see a patient with a minor problem that could have been dealt with during working hours, often weeks previously. This request for inconsequential night attention is not confined to the medical profession. 'Treble nine' calls to the police have increased by 25 per cent in two years, coinciding with the increase in GP call-outs, which have doubled in the same period.

Violence

Violence has been mentioned, but it has to be remembered that GPs are not infrequently assaulted and that every year or so a doctor is murdered. The murder of a doctor does not often stay in the headlines for long, almost as if the population accepts that medicine is a dangerous occupation and that there will be casualties. Recently, a GP was murdered and the murderer's family then proceeded to sue the estate of his victim for alleged shortcomings in the doctor's management of their relative's illness. The family was granted legal aid to pursue an untenable claim.

Violent patients are assigned to general practices. The doctor on whose list they are arbitrarily placed is obliged by the terms and conditions of their contract to provide 24-hour treatment or risk a complaint, which would be sustained. Police forces have advised that they cannot provide support for doctors in difficult situations, although many doctors have reason to be grateful to local police officers for support and help.

In a recent case, a patient was to be admitted to hospital under the Mental Health Act, but the doctor had reason to believe that the patient might have a shotgun in the house and might just be prepared to use it. The most senior police officer on duty that night informed the doctor that he would not allow his officers to intervene, as no offence had been committed. The psychiatric nursing shop-steward likewise declined to allow nurses from his trade union to enter the building. The GP convened a meeting in the local police station and a solution was rapidly agreed. The doctor was to go in first. If there was a gun and presumably a gunshot, or if there was any trouble, the others would rush to his assistance. The doctor's wife, who saw herself as a potential widow, was less than pleased. The entire event was stressful for all concerned.

GPs accept these events as being part and parcel of their working life, and inevitable when they are engaged with all members of our society, including criminals, the insane and the criminally insane. Stories of potential violence are related as jokes in medical circles, but doctors are well aware of the dangers they face and deal with them by making light of these situations.

Other problems

Doctors train to practise medicine, but their work requires them to become involved in events that have little to do with making people better. They inevitably have to appear in court as expert witnesses. The standard way in which attorneys deal with expert witnesses is to attempt to discredit them, as all doctors know. Appearances in court can be bruising and stressful. Committee work is another area in which doctors become involved and which can be quite alien to their training and interest. Public speaking is something that is hard for doctors to avoid; some find this difficult and stressful.

Community living

Some doctors work in a city environment and so are guaranteed some privacy, but the rural or small town GP is always conspicuous and will have, to a small extent, the problems of a celebrity. The doctor will be recognized and spoken to, and, as in so many jokes, consulted about medical problems in the filling station or at the village fête. They may begin to avoid local events because they have become traumatic.

Domestic stress

Stresses compound each other and, if the doctor experiences stress at home for personal or financial reasons, this is reflected in that doctor's professional life, and vice versa. Stresses accumulate and multiply. The doctor has to deal with all the stresses to which he or she is subject.

Dealing with stress

Doctors are prone to stress; that has been established. What do doctors do about it? They mostly do little or nothing until it is too late. Doctors rarely do anything routinely to mitigate the effects of stress in their everyday practice of medicine and in their ordinary lives. Domestic strife, divorce, irritability, aggression towards patients, staff and partners, and loss of professional competence, all proceed unchecked, when an admission of stress and attention to its management could make all the difference. GPs *do* know about stress; they can deal with it in others, so why do they not recognize it and deal with it in themselves?

Why do GPs not talk to their partners about stress? Why do they not confide in them? They prefer to adhere to a worn-out tradition of invulnerability long after other professionals facing traumatic situations have recognized the need for professional help. Why do doctors not recognize stress in their partners and give them the help they need? Perhaps the climate is not yet right for a sympathetic acceptance for the need for stress management in general practice, but that must change. If it is to change, what techniques are available, and what steps can be taken now to alleviate or pre-empt the stress that will result from the current attitudes to stress found in general practice?

Stress management techniques

The causes of GP stress are many and varied; there is therefore no simple all-embracing solution. The causes are subtle; often it is the small irritations, the inappropriate call-out, the sarcastic or caustic patient, that accumulate and annoy. The GP subjected to these situations will inevitably become stressed; of that there is no doubt. If that is the case, the personal measures for managing stress outlined in this book and explained in the appendices are relevant for doctors. When a GP feels stressed, there should be something he or she can do about it.

Doctors should learn and practise the relaxation exercises that they advocate and teach. This will not only allow them an understanding of what they are inviting their patients to do but give them a tool they can use to combat their own stress. The techniques, once learned, can be used between consultations if necessary, or in the car, or at night after a particularly frustrating and inappropriate call-out, so that some sleep may be possible and something salvaged from the night's activities.

As with patients, learning to relax gives early warning of increased tension and thus the opportunity of doing something about it. Proactive self-management of stress should be encouraged, not only for the individual but also for other interested members of the primary care team, including partners. Stress should be recognized and addressed. It should be discussed without embarrassment. If practice nurses or other health care professionals are teaching these techniques to patients, they should be encouraged to teach them first to other staff.

This demonstrates that the doctors understand and appreciate the stress that their employees experience. It also encourages a group awareness of stress; staff may come to have a better understanding of the stress under which doctors can be placed. Group practice of relaxation exercises leads to team building and may break down barriers between members of staff. Primarily, the acquisition of relaxation and breathing skills helps the individual doctor. The exercises are simple, easy to do, and they work. Why not practise them? Why not read the appendix or make a cassette and practise the exercises?

Recognizing the problem

Doctors should find it easy to identify the onset of stress. After all, they see it in others every day. They do not; doctors are the last to know. It is not possible to treat something you have not diagnosed, and no doctor will diagnose an illness that he or she has not thought of in the first place. Think stress; when things are going badly, think stress. Think, have I got it? Then think, what can I do about it? If you have practised the exercises, you will at least be as well off as your patients and you will know where to start.

Perhaps the doctor should spend time working out why there is stress. What are the reasons; what is going wrong? The cause may be obvious; it may be marital, but why? Is it, could it be, job-related? Almost certainly occupational stress is a contributing factor because general practice is a stressful occupation, so can the stresses be minimized?

Seeking support

Isolation causes stress; confiding helps stress. The doctor should confide his or her problems in a spouse, in a partner, in a health care professional, or in a doctors' stress management group, some of which are now becoming available. Seek help and advice, and act on that advice.

Nourish relationships

Doctors, stressed or otherwise, have emotional needs. The loss of the support of a spouse is devastating, but it is difficult for a spouse to be sympathetic if that opportunity is not given. A GP should share problems and worries and seek advice and emotional support. Isolation allows problems to get out of proportion. Medicine is only one part of a doctor's life and medical problems should be left in the consulting room as a matter of policy.

Physical well-being

Physical fitness, exercise and an interest away from medicine are of value. A doctor needs a brain holiday occasionally. Working at a fast pace locks the mind on to the job. That works for a short time but, in the longer term, it is very destructive and it is imperative that a doctor should develop outside interests.

Administration and planning

Perhaps unexpectedly, research by Howie *et al.* (1992) suggest that more mundane factors contribute substantially to stress in doctors. Poor organization and planning leading to surgeries that overrun, permit interruptions or allow the doctor to work after a night on call contribute greatly to stress. Pressure of work, large personal list sizes, and a lack of planning or of managing administrative work must also contribute.

Howie *et al.* demonstrated that, the longer a surgery ran and the longer patients had to wait to see the doctor, the higher was the stress for that doctor. Yet many doctors start their surgeries more than 10 minutes late, often for the best of reasons, but with the most disastrous of results. If a doctor knows that patients are waiting for more than 10 minutes, the stress rate rises in a linear fashion. Nonappointment surgeries are more stressful than appointment surgeries, and a run of difficult patients does not help. Matching the appointment system to one's rate of consultation is of paramount importance, so are starting on time and avoiding interruptions. Allow breaks; allow time to adjust between patients, particularly if one has been especially difficult.

Sharing problems

GPs are loners, they work by themselves. Social workers, nurses and most other professional health workers have line managers and group responsibility. The essence of general practice is that the patient knows that the relationship with the doctor is strictly one-to-one, and that it is as private as the confessional. Some information is committed to paper, and some is typed by secretaries, but the core of the conversation is private. That places a great burden on the confidant, the doctor. The doctor has no line manager requiring a detailed report, no confessor. Doctors attending meetings with social workers or others know how public private information can be. The doctor keeps his or her counsel, but at a cost.

This is a cost that doctors should not have to pay. It is important that they should share problems, even if it is just over coffee. There should be time in a working day for the exchange of concerns. Doctors in a practice should strive to share the load. The structure for doing this needs to be built into the day's schedule in the form of informal meetings and coffee breaks.

General practitioner stress groups

There is some interest in stress management groups for GPs, but some groups that have been started have had to discontinue because of poor support. GPs by and large have been slow to become involved in this activity, which is intended to pre-empt stress-related problems. Stress is still not admitted as a problem for doctors and there will have to be a change in attitudes before such public stress prophylaxis is acceptable.

Night work

Call-outs have doubled in general practice over a few years, as has public expectation of the service provided by doctors. It simply is not possible to work by day *and* night. It is exhausting and erodes professional competence as well as personal relationships. Ways have to be found to manage the 24-hour commitment to allow a doctor time to rest and relax, and to be with his or her family.

Women general practitioners

Women GPs fare less well than their male colleagues when it comes to stress. Combining part-time work with a home commitment is the most stressful of all. Black female part-time doctors experience the most stress. This is a problem that the profession as a whole has to consider as the percentage of women in practice increases. Provision will have to be made for part-time GPs, taking the stressful nature of the job into account.

Check list

When a doctor is feeling unwell, psychological problems should be considered. A doctor might ask: 'Am I depressed? Do I feel sad? Is my mood low? Am I tearful? Do I have problems with coping?' If a doctor is depressed, it is important that help is sought immediately.

A doctor might also wish to consider the possibility of a stress-related problem and work through a check list:

- Am I tired all the time?
- Do I sleep well?
- Do I wake with a sore neck and sore jaw muscles?
- Do I wake with nail marks on the palms of my hands from fist clenching?
- Do I have problems with coping during the day?
- Are my relationships breaking down?

If stress is a problem, wonder why. Why am I under so much pressure?

- Am I trying to do too much?
- Have I too many commitments?
- Am I letting things slip?
- Do I start my surgeries on time?
- Do my surgeries run to time?
- Do I deal adequately with problem patients?
- Do I manage my time successfully?

If a doctor is suffering from occupational stress, often aggravated by domestic or personal stress, how can this be tackled? Clearly, what is right for patients is right for their doctors. Everything in this book is as relevant to the management of a doctor's stress as it is to a patient's stress.

Summary

- General practice is stressful.
- GPs are slow to admit that the may be vulnerable to stress.
- GPs are slow to seek help.
- The medical profession is slow to provide such help.
- GPs should be prepared to treat their own stress.
- GPs should look for stress in colleagues and offer help.
- GPs should look at ways of managing their practice to enable the reduction of stress.

Appendices

Guidelines for doctors and clerical workers for producing written material for patients

Most doctors have access to the assistance of a clerical worker who has the use of word processing facilities. Such facilities can easily be used to produce very professional-looking information for patients. The basic text for written relaxation instructions and for a booklet on stress are provided in Appendices 4 and 5.

It is especially useful to add to the booklet some information about the support that is available locally, both statutory and from other community groups and services. This can be collated fairly easily in most areas. You can also include any of the more general 'Useful addresses' given in Appendix 6 that seem relevant.

Here is some further guidance:

What size should the leaflet be?

- Arrange the material in a way that makes photocopying or printing easy to do using the resources available.
- Make the leaflet a size that is easy for the patient to take home in a pocket or a bag.
- If it can only easily be produced in A4 format or is too big for a pocket, provide a fairly stout plain envelope. Most patients will not want to be seen carrying a stress management leaflet, and it can also be easily damaged if not protected from the elements.

What is the best size of type?

- The best size for most patients will be 12-point type. If it is easy to do so, a larger type could be provided for those with poor eyesight.

What about the font?

- Choose a font that looks professional but friendly, preferably not one that looks as if a typewriter has been used. 'Times New Roman' or 'Arial' are suitable and easily available. Keep to one font throughout.

What is the best way to set it out?

An example of a page from a leaflet is shown in Appendix 8. Here are some useful pointers to make a leaflet attractive and easy to read:

- Do not cram the material into the pages. This puts the reader off. Space it out well, with good margins.
- Justify only to the left-hand margin.
- Start the headings on the left-hand margin, not in the centre, as this is easier to read.
- Make the headings stand out by using space around them or by making them bold or a larger size of type (as in this book).
- Use bold or italic for emphasis, but use this sparingly as it can be distracting and confusing.
- Do not use capitals or underlining for headings or emphasis, as this is very distracting for the reader.
- Do not hyphenate words at the end of a line.
- Lists can be produced in columns in either a box or table to make them easier to read.

What about coloured paper?

- This can be a useful addition, but choose pale colours such as cream, green or lemon.

Should illustrations be added?

These are not essential, but if available, a few simple well-chosen illustrations or graphics can break up the text, add to understanding, and make the leaflet more readable:

- Make them simple and easily understood in relation to the text.
- Keep their size in proportion to their connection with the text.
- Do not use humour or cartoons unless you have a great deal of experience of dealing with stress, as this is a serious subject for patients and it is very easy to hit the wrong note.
- Do not fit the text around the graphics, as this is difficult to read.
- Make sure no patient group is excluded or emphasized – stress can happen to anyone.

Guidelines for doctors for producing an audio cassette of relaxation instructions

Using the text provided in Appendix 3, it is really very straightforward and inexpensive to produce a relaxation cassette of reasonable quality for patient use. Once it is prepared, simply keep several master copies in your surgery, and loan them to the patient to copy and return. A C90 tape is a good length, as it leaves plenty of space for patients to add their favourite relaxing music or other relaxing sounds if they wish.

- Use your own voice, or that of one of your friends or colleagues.
- The kind of voice does not really matter as long as it can easily be understood, and it carries warmth and reassurance.
- Use a good quality cassette recorder with or without a free-standing microphone.
- Before the actual recording, practise recording part of the text to get used to it.
- Simply read the text very slowly in a very calming voice, leaving appropriate gaps when the patient has to do something. Speak warmly and reassuringly. It helps if you imagine you are talking directly to a patient, or if you have someone to follow the instructions as you talk.
- Set the text out in front of you where you can read it without rustling or turning pages and still speak into the microphone. If you are using an in-built microphone, speak directly into it.
- Avoid speaking in a monotone.
- Play back your practice run to check you have got the speed and tone right, and that you have left enough time for the patient to follow the instructions. Have as many practice runs as you need.
- Read the whole text through without recording, to check out and practise any areas over which you might stumble.
- For your final recording, choose a time and a place where there are no background noises or distractions. If you have access to a recording studio, so much the better, but that would usually be expensive.

- Read each section of text, including the headings, very slowly in a very calm voice, leaving gaps when the patient has to do something. Leave a long gap between tracks. If you can stop the recording silently between tracks, you can have a break then.
- Alter the wording if needed to suit your own personal style.
- Test the recording out on a volunteer before putting it to general use.

Other useful additions:

- Patients often express a preference for a male or female voice on the tape, so, if you have the time or the opportunity, you could record one of each.
- An appropriate translation of the text can be used for patients from ethnic minority groups.

Appendix 3

Labelling and text for relaxation audio cassette

Labelling

'Relaxation'

Side One: Introduction
Total Relaxation
Side Two: Introduction
Three Types of Rapid Relaxation
Partial Relaxation
WARNING: This cassette must not be played whilst driving or operating machinery.

Text (Instructions to the doctor or other speaker are in italics.)

Side One

Track 1: Introduction
This tape contains instructions for three types of relaxation. Please remember that you should not play this tape if you are driving, operating machinery or in charge of other people or children. And remember not to get up suddenly whilst using the tape, as you may feel slightly dizzy. Use a quiet room where you won't be disturbed, take the phone off the hook, and ignore the doorbell. Always allow enough time for you to become fully alert again after you've used the tape, before you go back to your usual activities.

On this side of the tape, Side One, there are instructions for total relaxation. This is the first stage in learning to relax. You should allow around 30 minutes for this, and try to practise every day. Try this out when you're already feeling quite relaxed until you get the hang of it. Choose a time when you're not too tired, or you may fall asleep. Space has been left after this track for you to add your own favourite relaxing music or other sounds if this would be helpful.

After a few weeks, if you are relaxing well with these instructions, you can move on to Side Two. This second side has instructions for three techniques of rapid relaxation. Each of these allows you to relax very quickly. You should try out these three methods, and choose those that suit you best for when you need to relax quickly. You can still be using total relaxation any time you feel like it.

Also on Side Two there are instructions for partial relaxation. This helps you to be able to use parts of your body (for example, your hands for writing, or while you are talking to people) and yet keep the remainder of your body as relaxed as possible. You should begin by practising only total relaxation, until you feel it is working for you. You should then move on to the other techniques.

None of these techniques is in any way strenuous, but if you are in any doubt about your fitness to carry them out safely, then listen first to the instructions, and check with your doctor if you're still unsure.

Relaxation, like any other skill, takes time to learn, so don't expect too much too soon, and don't try too hard; this will only increase your tension. Simply listen and allow the relaxation to happen on its own. You may even find to begin with that you can only relax fleetingly before tension returns, or your mind begins to wander. Don't be concerned about this, simply return your thoughts to my voice and continue as instructed. With practice, you will find that you relax more and more deeply and efficiently. In time, you should also be able to practise these techniques without the tape to help you, so that you can use them anywhere and any time that you need them.

Track 2: Total relaxation
Lie or sit with your head supported, with your arms by your side and your legs uncrossed. Make sure that your clothing is loose, and that you are warm and comfortable. You should allow at least half an hour for this session, and remember to make sure you are fully alert again before going about your usual activities.

I want you now to pay attention to your breathing. Just become aware of your breathing, and allow it to slow down, just a little bit. If you can, breathe in through your nose and out through your mouth. If that is difficult, just breathe in a way in which you feel comfortable. Slowly sigh out each breath, letting your shoulders drop. Feel the tension beginning to leave your body. Each time you breathe out, think of the word PEACE ... PEACE ... PEACE.

Now bring your attention to your fingers and your hands. Clench the fists of both your hands, tight ... hold them tight ... feel the tension ... (*all muscle groups should be tensed for around five or six seconds altogether*) ... now, let that tension go and relax them completely.

Now your arms: bring your thoughts to your arms. Straighten up both arms tightly, tighter, feel the tension up and down your arms .... Now let that tension go, let them become heavier and heavier as they relax completely.

Notice how your breathing is becoming more and more relaxed. Sigh away the tension as you breathe out, think of the word PEACE ... PEACE ....

Bring your attention now to your shoulders. Hunch up your shoulders, feel the tension ... tighter .... Now let that tension go, let them sink deeper and deeper, and become more and more relaxed.

Now your face and your head: screw up your face, your eyes, your nose, your mouth, clench your teeth, lift your head a little from its support, feel all of that tension .... Now let it go, let it all go, draining away from your body. Let your head grow heavier and heavier, and sink deeper and deeper, becoming more and more relaxed. Allow your jaw to sag and your mouth to open slightly. Enjoy the feeling of relaxation. Breathe slowly and evenly, in through your nose and out through your mouth, if you can, letting your stomach, your lower chest and then your upper chest rise as you breathe in, and then fall as you breathe out. PEACE ... PEACE ... PEACE ....

Now move your attention to your stomach and your back. Pull in the muscles of your stomach and of your bottom. Pull them in tight, tighter ..., now relax them. Let that tension go, draining away as you become heavier and heavier, and more and more relaxed. Breathe slowly and evenly. PEACE ... PEACE .... Each time you breathe out, feel the tension draining from your upper chest, your stomach and your back. PEACE ... PEACE .... Enjoy the feeling of relaxation. Now arch your back slightly. Hold it... now let the tension go, draining away from your back. Enjoy that feeling of relaxation.

Now your legs and your feet: point each foot, curl up your toes, and straighten each leg tight, tighter. Hold it ... feel the tension .... Now let it all go. Let it drain away as your legs and your whole body grow heavier and heavier and more relaxed. Feel yourself sinking deeper, and deeper and becoming more and more relaxed. Enjoy this feeling of complete relaxation. Concentrate on the word PEACE, or on a pleasant scene that you find calming or soothing: a warm beach, a sunny country scene, or the warm glow of a fire. Enjoy these feelings for a few moments. (*Allow around a minute here.*)

Now bring your thoughts back to your body. Slowly become more alert. Have a yawn and a stretch if you feel like it, but don't get up too quickly. You can now either continue relaxing with some music or other sounds, which you can add to the tape, or, in your own time and without rushing, gently sit up and, when you feel alert, return to your usual activities.

Side Two

Track 1: Introduction
Three techniques for rapid relaxation, and one for partial relaxation will follow. The rapid relaxation methods all help you to relax very quickly, in a few minutes or even less. Practise with each of these, and try partial relaxation to find out which methods are best suited to your needs.

Before practising with this side of the cassette, you should feel that you are relaxing well with total relaxation on Side One. Once mastered, these techniques may be used to help you in everyday life without the help of the tape. You can still be using total relaxation any time you feel like it.

Track 2: Rapid relaxation, technique one
This is simply a speeded up version of total relaxation. You can do this almost anywhere and at any time. With practice, it can be done in seconds.

- Lie or sit, and allow your breathing to slow down. Breathe in through your nose and out through your mouth, thinking PEACE ... each time you breathe out. Breathe slowly and evenly.

- Now tense your hands and your arms, tight ... tight ... (*allow five or six seconds tensing each time*). Keep your breathing at ease. Let the tension start to leave your body. Now hunch up your shoulders and tighten the muscles in your face, scalp and neck ... hold it ... now let go ... let the tension drain away. Breathe slowly and evenly. Now pull in your stomach and your bottom tightly ... then let them all go. Breathe easily ... PEACE .... Lastly, your feet and legs: point your toes, tense up your legs tightly ... now let go. Let the relaxation take over completely as all the tension disappears. Allow your whole body to become more and more relaxed and at PEACE .... Enjoy this feeling of relaxation for a few moments. (*Allow at least one minute here.*)

- Now, slowly rouse yourself. Have a yawn and a stretch and slowly sit up. In your own time, once you are fully alert, go back to your usual activities.

Track 3: Rapid relaxation, technique two
This again can be done at any time, anywhere, the moment you feel tension developing. With practice, it can be done in seconds.

Slow down your breathing. Breathe in through your nose and out through your mouth if you can. Think of the word PEACE each time you breathe out. Breathe slowly and evenly.

Now tense all of your body at the same time: hands clenched, arms and shoulders tight, face, head, neck, chest, stomach, legs and feet all tense. Hold them all tightly for a few seconds … now let it all go … let it all drain away, far away from your body. Let the relaxation and the peace take over entirely, all through your body from the tips of your fingers to your toes. Breathe slowly and evenly. PEACE … PEACE …. Enjoy the relaxation and then, in your own time, rouse yourself and return to your usual activities as soon as you are fully alert.

Track 4: Rapid relaxation, technique three
This method takes a little more practice, but there is no need to tense up your muscles. It can be done in seconds, and nobody will even be aware you are doing it.

Slow down your breathing. Breathe in through your nose and out through your mouth if you can. Think of the word PEACE each time you breathe out. Breathe slowly and evenly. Now concentrate on your fingers and hands. Don't tense them. Simply concentrate on letting them relax completely. Imagining them growing heavier and warmer will help. Let all the tension go from your hands.

Now concentrate on your arms and your shoulders. Let the tension drain away from them and let them relax completely: very heavy, very relaxed.

Now let the tension drain away from your neck, your face and your head. Let it all go. They are feeling very heavy and very relaxed. Your stomach and your back are relaxing now. Let the tension go from them, as you grow heavier and heavier and more and more relaxed. Breathe slowly and evenly, letting the relaxation deepen. Your legs and your feet: let the tension drain away from them too and let the relaxation take over your entire body.

You are now feeling heavier and more and more relaxed, sinking deeper and deeper. PEACE … PEACE …. Enjoy the relaxation for a few moments, and then, in your own time, rouse yourself, and, when you are fully alert, return to your usual activities.

Track 5: Partial relaxation
Before practising this type of relaxation, you should already be completely relaxed. Perhaps a good time is after a session of total or rapid relaxation.

There are obviously times when your body cannot be entirely relaxed. Imagine driving, walking, or even just talking, with all of your muscles totally relaxed. Impossible: but practising partial relaxation will help you to keep any unnecessary muscle tension to a minimum while you are involved in any of these or other activities.

You should already be relaxed, so concentrate for a moment on your breathing. Breathe slowly and evenly, and think of the word PEACE … each time you breathe out.

Now slowly raise your hands and start slowly to make some of your everyday hand movements. You might pretend to be driving, typing, stirring a pot, writing or whatever, but, while you are doing this, try to allow the rest of your body to stay totally relaxed: no tension anywhere. Practise this for a few moments, concentrating on keeping the rest of your body relaxed and free of tension. Get to know this feeling of partial relaxation, so that you can bring it into your everyday life. Now place your hands back by your sides and relax your body completely ... (*slight pause here*).

Slowly open your eyes and say a few words: your name and address, or something about the weather, or just count slowly upwards from one. Concentrate on keeping the rest of your body totally relaxed and free of tension. Practise this for a few moments. Get to know this feeling of partial relaxation. Now close your eyes and allow yourself to relax completely again ... (*slight pause here*).

Now slowly reopen your eyes, and, in your own time without rushing, gradually sit up. Breathe slowly and evenly, and think of the word PEACE ... each time you breathe out. Make sure there is no unnecessary tension anywhere in your body. Get to know this feeling of sitting in a totally relaxed way. Remember how it feels. Now, once again, in your own time, gradually stand up, and just stand for a few moments, making sure there is no extra tension anywhere other than what you need to stand up. Feel what it is like to stand in a totally relaxed way ....

Next slowly take a few steps round the room, keeping as relaxed as possible, with no more tension than is needed to walk. Get to know the feeling so that you can use it in everyday life whenever you might need it.

Now gradually sit or lie down again, and let go completely. Relax your body totally, breathe slowly and evenly, and, each time you breathe out, think PEACE ... PEACE ....

Enjoy the relaxation for a few moments, then, in your own time and without rushing, slowly rouse yourself and, when you are fully alert again, return to your usual activities.

Appendix 4

Written relaxation instructions for patients

(These are an alternative to a relaxation audio cassette and can be given with or without the patient booklet.)

Introduction and guidelines

This leaflet contains instructions for three types of relaxation. Please remember that you should not practise these if you are driving, operating machinery or in charge of other people or children. And remember not to get up suddenly whilst using the instructions, as you may feel slightly dizzy. Use a quiet room where you won't be disturbed, take the phone off the hook, and ignore the doorbell. Keep your eyes open to read the instructions until you can remember them, then close your eyes. Always allow enough time for you to become fully alert again after you've practised, before you go back to your usual activities.

First, you will find instructions for total relaxation. This is the first stage in learning to relax. You should allow around 30 minutes for this, and try to practise every day. Try this out when you're already feeling quite relaxed until you get the hang of it. Choose a time when you're not too tired, or you may fall asleep.

After a few weeks, if you are relaxing well with these instructions, you can move on to the three techniques of rapid relaxation. Each of these allows you to relax very quickly. You should try out these three methods, and choose those that suit you best for when you need to relax quickly. You can still be using total relaxation any time you feel like it.

After this, there are instructions for partial relaxation. This helps you to be able to use parts of your body (for example, your hands for writing, or while you are talking to people), and yet keep the remainder of your body as relaxed as possible. You should begin by practising only total relaxation, until you feel it is working for you. You should then move on to the other techniques.

None of these techniques is in any way strenuous, but if you are in any doubt about your fitness to carry them out safely, then first read the instructions, and check with your doctor if you're still unsure.

Relaxation, like any other skill, takes time to learn, so don't expect too much too soon, and don't try too hard; this will only increase your tension. Simply listen and allow the relaxation to happen on its own.

You may even find to begin with that you can only relax fleetingly before tension returns, or your mind begins to wander. Don't be concerned about this, simply return to what you were doing and continue as instructed. With practice, you will find that you relax more and more deeply and efficiently. In time, you should also be able to practise these techniques without the instructions to help you, so that you can use them anywhere and any time that you need them.

Total relaxation

(*Allow at least 30 minutes.*)

- Lie on your back, or sit up in a comfortable chair, preferably with some support for your head. Carry out the following very, very slowly ....

- Breathe slowly and evenly for a few moments, allowing yourself to unwind a little bit with each outward breath. Now clench your fists and hold them really tightly for five or six seconds. Feel the tension. Now release them suddenly. Let all the tension go, and relax them completely. You may notice a feeling of warmth and heaviness in your fingers, hands and lower arms. These are an important sign that you are relaxing properly.

- Now, hunch up your shoulders. Feel that tension. Hold it for five or six seconds. Now let your shoulders slump suddenly. Feel the relief. Let your breathing slow even further. Now push your head back a little, tensing your neck. Feel the tension. Now let your head return to its position, and relax ....

- Next, frown and close your eyes tightly, purse your lips, clench your jaws and press your tongue against the roof of your mouth. Feel all sorts of tension in your head and face. Hold it. Now suddenly let it all go. Let your jaw sag and your mouth open slightly. Breathe slowly and evenly. Enjoy the feelings of relaxation.

- Now arch your back slightly. Hold it. Now relax. Enjoy that relaxation.

- Pull in your stomach hard, harder. Now let it go. Breathe slowly and evenly. Enjoy the feelings of relaxation.

- Point your toes away from you, and curl your toes under, tightly. Feel the tension throughout your legs. Hold it ... now suddenly let go and relax again. Let even more tension go as you breathe out.

- Your whole body will now feel heavy and completely relaxed. Your breathing will be slow and gentle. Allow yourself to feel heavier and heavier, and more and more relaxed. Enjoy these feelings for a few moments, or longer if you have the time.

- When you feel ready, finish your session gradually. In your own time, with no rush, allow yourself to become more alert. Have a yawn and a stretch if you feel like it.
- When you feel fully alert, return to what you were doing.

Rapid relaxation

Here are three methods. Try them all, allowing 5–10 minutes for each, and find out which ones suit you best.

Method one
Lie or sit comfortably, and allow your breathing to become slow and even. Now concentrate on your hands and arms. Don't tense them. Just concentrate on allowing all the tension to drain away from them. Continue concentrating like this on each part of your body in turn, in the same order as for total relaxation – hands and arms, shoulders, neck and head, face, back and stomach, legs and feet – letting all the tension drain away, without tensing them first. Enjoy the feeling of relaxation you have produced for a few moments, or more if you have time, then finish your session as for total relaxation.

Method two
Follow the instructions as for total relaxation, but speed up the whole process, so that you can become relaxed within a minute or two. Finish off as before.

Method three
Lie or sit comfortably, allowing your breathing to become slow and regular. Now, all at the same time, deliberately tense up tightly, your whole body, and hold it for a few seconds – hands, arms, shoulders, neck and head, face, back and stomach, legs and feet – then suddenly let it all go and allow relaxation to take over. Repeat the whole process once more if necessary. Enjoy the relaxation for a few moments, or longer if you have time, then finish off your session as before.

Partial relaxation

Make sure that you are already completely relaxed before you try this type of relaxation. The idea is to be able to learn to relax the remainder of your body whilst using part of it. You should allow 10–15 minutes. Here is what to do:

- Lie or sit, totally relaxed, for a few moments.
- Now raise your hands, and begin moving them in the air as if you are

writing, typing or carrying out some other relevant action. Try to keep the rest of your body completely relaxed as you do this. Continue doing this for a few moments.

- Now, with your eyes open, look around the room, keeping your head still. Move your eyes only, and again, try to keep the rest of your body relaxed and at ease.

- Now look around further by moving your head a little, again, keeping the rest of your body relaxed. Now keep your head and eyes still, and try saying a few words, again keeping your body relaxed. Now relax completely again for a few moments.

- Next, sit up slowly, and practise sitting up with your eyes open, totally relaxed for a few moments. Keep your whole body relaxed and at ease.

- Now, very slowly stand up and see if you can stand in a relaxed way, with no more tension than required. After standing still for a few moments, walk around a little, pick something up and carry it, then replace it – all the time keeping relaxed any part of your body not in use. Use only the minimum of tension in the muscles that you are using.

- Now, gradually lie or sit down again, and relax your whole body once more. Allow any tension to drain away, and enjoy the feeling of complete relaxation for a few moments, or more if you have time.

- Finish the session as before.

Text for a comprehensive patient booklet to accompany a relaxation cassette or written relaxation instructions

(Guidelines on setting this out are given in Appendix 1. Remember to leave empty space at the end for the progress diary.)

How to cope better with stress

What is this booklet for?

You have been given this booklet because you are experiencing some unpleasant effects of stress. This can happen to anyone at all and is very common these days. There is no magic pill for this, and common sense doesn't have much to offer for coping with stress. So this booklet aims to explain more about what is happening to you, and suggest straight-forward things you can do for yourself to make you feel better. You should also have been given a cassette or a leaflet containing relaxation instructions. Start using the relaxation instructions every day, and begin working through this booklet at your own pace, ticking or highlighting anything you think would be helpful for you. You can use the diary at the back to keep tabs on your progress.

Remember that, although this booklet is not a prescription, it is just as important as one.

Understanding stress

What is stress?
At its simplest, people feel stressed when the pressure of circumstances makes them feel one or more of the following:

- Threatened
- Unsure or unfamiliar
- Overwhelmed
- Trapped
- Dissatisfied or unhappy

- That they can't cope as well as they want to
- That they can't cope at all.

Depending on the particular circumstances, stress like this can be short-lasting, or go on for months or even years. Stress causes a range of usually unpleasant symptoms, which can undermine our overall health and well-being.

Some possible causes of your stress
Here are some examples of what may be causing you to feel the way you do:

- Losing your job
- Being unemployed
- Housing problems
- Money problems
- Caring for young children
- Relationship difficulties (partner, children, parents, neighbours ...)
- Being a carer (for a person who is elderly, mentally ill, disabled, etc.)
- Having too much or too little to do
- Being ill, or caring for someone who is ill
- You or someone you care about is having a drink or a drugs problem
- Someone you care about is having problems
- Constant daily hassles
- Problems at work (lack of control, overloaded, under-valued, etc.)
- Business worries
- Lots of small, or several large, changes in your life over a recent period (up to several years or more)
- Accident, loss or bereavement
- Being faced with particular situations that you find difficult (speaking in public, depending on other people, working as a team ...)
- Nothing in particular, just lots of things adding up.

Having said that, stress is not always connected with bad things. Even happy events, such as a wedding, the birth of a baby, or a new house, can be just as stressful. In fact, we all need a certain amount of challenge in our lives, but if this gets too much for us, we feel stressed.

How stress makes you feel
Stress upsets our normal body chemistry and produces all sorts of symptoms. If you have not already been seen by your doctor, who might

have confirmed that your symptoms are the result of stress, do so as soon as you can. Here are some of the signs and symptoms of stress. You may be experiencing one or more of these:

- Physical:
  - Headaches
  - Indigestion/churning stomach
  - Palpitations
  - Difficulty with taking a deep breath
  - Difficulty with swallowing
  - Nausea
  - Tiredness;
  - Aches and pains
  - Muscle twitches
  - Sweating
  - Muscle tension
  - Weight gain or loss
  - Trembling
  - Dry mouth
  - Tingling in fingers, toes or face.

- Emotional:
  - Irritability
  - Forgetfulness
  - Panicky
  - Gloomy thoughts
  - Fearfulness
  - Anxiety/worry
  - Depression
  - Negative thinking
  - Feeling 'unreal'.

- Behavioural:
  - Nail biting
  - Restlessness
  - Agitation
  - Can't sleep or very sleepy
  - Eating too much or too little
  - Making mistakes
  - Poor concentration
  - change in usual behaviour
  - Indecision
  - Anger
  - Forgetfulness
  - Increased smoking, or drinking.

Panic attacks

Sometimes stress can cause people to have attacks of particularly acute anxiety, called panic attacks. Their stomach churns, their heart races, their breathing may be rapid, and they may sweat, feel faint, feel overwhelming fear, panic and a sense of impending disaster, along with a pressing need to escape from the situation in which they find themselves.

Such attacks are actually the body's normal reaction to threat or danger, brought into action by the automatic part of the nervous system. This is meant to prepare the body to fight the source of the danger, or run away from it, but, in today's world, this is no help to us. Threats and dangers such as mounting bills or overwork cannot be dealt with in this way, so all of this mobilization simply has no outlet and makes us feel awful instead. This means that panic attacks will do you no actual harm at all. If they are a problem for you, some practical tips on dealing with them are given later.

Breathing

Even the lowest level of stress can increase your rate of breathing, and long-term or severe stress can disrupt normal breathing entirely. These kinds of changes in your breathing over long periods of time can upset the normal body chemistry, and can cause many of the symptoms already mentioned, including panic, feeling faint, tingling and poor concentration.

There are no overnight miracle cures

If you really put into action the advice offered to you here, you should find a great improvement, but don't be discouraged if there is no immediate response. This takes time to happen; it may take anything from a few days or weeks, to some months or more. You may also find that you have ups and downs. Keeping notes in the Progress Diary at the back of this booklet helps you to see how you are progressing overall. If you feel sure that you are not progressing as you should, have another word with your GP, who may be able to refer you for further help.

Cassette tape on loan

Remember, if you have received a cassette tape from your doctor, this is likely to be on loan, and you should return it for someone else to use after you've made your own copy.

What about my medication?

If you have been taking medication for stress, do not make changes to this without medical advice. If after some time you are feeling better, discuss with your doctor the possibility of gradually reducing your medication.

How your partner, family or friends can help
Some partners, families or friends are more supportive than others. If you feel you know someone who will be supportive, let them read this booklet. This will help them to understand what you are trying to do, and to see that you will need support and encouragement and the time and space to practise new skills such as relaxation.

Where do I go from here?
All of the ten tips given later fall into two main categories:

• Doing something about the cause or causes of the stress;
• Cushioning yourself from the impact of the stress.

Here's where to start:

• Start to practise relaxation immediately and every day.
• Read the ten tips that follow, and tick or highlight the suggestions that you think might apply to you. Start these off one at a time, rather than all at once. If you try to make too many changes at once, you'll feel more stressed, and never keep it up. As soon as one change is established, you're ready for the next one.
• Use the Progress Diary at the back of this booklet to keep tabs on how things are going.
• Try to get copies of some of the books or cassettes listed at the end of this booklet, the ones that you think might help. Common sense doesn't have much to offer for coping with stress.
• Let your doctor know how things are going, and talk to him or her if you're having problems.

Ten practical tips

1. Can you do anything about the cause of your stress?
You may now have some idea of what is causing your stress, and your first step is to decide whether you can actually do something about this cause:

• *If you think you can.* Perhaps you need to seek out expert advice or support on how to deal with the problem, but, one way or another, sort it out. Follow the other nine tips to help you to cope while you do this.

- *If you're sure you can't.* Do all you can to cushion yourself from its effects, using the rest of this leaflet to tell you how.
- *If you're not sure.* Seek out expert advice and support to help to clarify the situation. Use this leaflet to help you in the meantime.

If you are still unsure of the cause of your stress, it is probably being caused by your lifestyle or general approach to life. The tips that follow may help sort this out.

Having begun to think about what you can do about the stress itself, what else can you do?

2. Slow down and make time for relaxation

There are all sorts of ways to relax; it's down to your preferences. The important thing is that you should allow your body to slow down and relax completely at least once every day. A lazy bath, a walk, a visit to friends, music, yoga, sport, and so on. Relaxation exercises are useful because you can usually fit them into your day, and they are also helpful to use to keep stress under control in problem situations. With practice, you should be able to relax in just a few minutes, or even less.

Using your audio cassette or written instructions, you should begin by practising the methods given every day until they begin to work for you. Then you can use them as a regular relaxing break, to help you to cope better with those difficult situations.

It is sometimes useful to join a relaxation group in your area, especially if it's hard to get the time and space at home. Yoga classes are another option as they usually end with a relaxation session.

If your time is tight, you may think that taking time out to do this will just get you even further behind, but this is not the case. If your body is allowed to relax regularly, you will actually be able to get more done more effectively with the time left, because you are refreshed and energized.

You can also relax your mind as follows:

- Slow down and relax your body.
- Once relaxed, picture as clearly as you can, or focus your mind on any one of these:
  - Waves lapping on the sea-shore
  - Branches swaying in the breeze
  - Deep dark green velvet
  - A word or phrase such as 'peace', 'calm', 'relax'
  - A calming poem, prayer or picture.

3. Think about your breathing

Breathing normally can help to relieve many of the symptoms of stress, and will also help you to cope better in stressful situations. Breathing techniques are also an alternative way to relax. Here is a simple technique to help you to slow and regulate your breathing, yet still remain alert:

- Lie down or sit with good support.
- Let your breath go, then take a gentle breath in, to your own slow silent count of 1 ... 2 ... 3 ..., then breathe out in your own time, again to your own slow and silent count of 1 ... 2 ... 3.
- Continue breathing gently to this rhythm for a few minutes.
- With practice, you will be able to leave out the counting, and just go into this rhythm when you have the need.

4. Take regular breaks
- Managing your time:
  - Take regular breaks, especially from a stressful situation; suitably refreshed, you will be able to cope better and work more efficiently on your return; even a five-minute break in a stressful morning can work wonders.
  - Make time for yourself, and for hobbies, interests and leisure pursuits; this takes your mind off your troubles, and helps to keep them in perspective.
  - If you have too much time on your hands, get involved in a hobby or a voluntary activity, preferably with other people.
  - Regularly do things that you enjoy.
- If time is tight:
  - Keep lists of jobs to be done, separating the urgent from the non-urgent.
  - Select and prioritize what you do: you can't do it all.
  - Plan your days and weeks in advance and keep a diary.
  - Be organized and know where everything is.
  - Do one job at a time.
  - Delegate whenever possible.

5. Help yourself with your lifestyle
Here are some general tips. Remember to tick or highlight those that you think apply to you, and make changes one at a time, with your Progress Diary to help you to keep track.

- General:
  - Eat a well-balanced diet, low in sugar, salt and fat, and high in fibre.
  - Don't skip meals, especially breakfast and lunch.

- Avoid food or drink containing caffeine (e.g. cola, coffee, chocolate).
- Do not use alcohol or other substances to help you to sleep or relax.
- Bear in mind the recommended weekly alcohol intake if you do drink.
- Get plenty of restful sleep; use relaxation or breathing techniques if you can't get off to sleep, or if you wake up during the night.

• Exercise:
- Regular physical activity that you enjoy and that fits in with your lifestyle is a very good cushion for stress.
- Walking is generally all right for most people, but if you're unsure about beginning or resuming a particular form of exercise, check with your doctor first.
- A contact sport is particularly useful if you are suppressing anger or frustration due to work or some other situation.

6. Coping with panic attacks

If you have panic attacks, the key is to catch them early, and stop them in their tracks. This puts you back in control. Here is one way of doing this. Don't be put off if this method doesn't work the first or even the second time you try it. Keep at it; it can be very effective:

Work out what are your own first signs of a panic attack. This might be a lurch in the stomach, a thought in your mind, your heart rate rising, or something else you've noticed. Look out for these first signs, and when you notice them, you should immediately:

Pause ... and make yourself comfortable (sit down, lean on something etc.).
Absorb ... details of what's going on around you.
Use ... any method of relaxing quickly that works well for you, then,
Slowly ... when you feel better.
Ease ... yourself back into what you were doing.

That's:

P   Pause,
A   Absorb details around you,
U   Use relaxation, then
S   Slowly,
E   Ease yourself back ....

7. Watch out for your thinking style

This may sound trendy or unusual, but being aware of some of the ways that your thinking can be contributing to your stress can make a real difference. Once you're aware of it, you're half way to changing it. We all know people who seem to be able to cope with anything. The difference is usually in their attitude to life. Here are some ideas to think about. Tick or highlight anything that might apply to you:

- Avoid negative thinking:
  - Don't ignore the ordinary or good things that happen each day as if they don't count for some reason. Take account of the bad side of life, but don't dwell on it.
  - When things go wrong, it's not always your fault. Other people or just the situation are just as often to blame.
  - Take your mind off your problems as much as you can. They grow bigger the more you concentrate on them.
- Avoid 'should', 'ought' and 'must' thinking:
  - Do you often find yourself using one of these words, 'I must do this', 'I ought to do that', and so on?
  - Ask yourself who is setting these personal standards and targets, and whether you are setting them too high.
  - Let yourself off the hook, and lower these standards if necessary.
- Mistaken beliefs: Your whole thinking may have at its heart one or more mistaken assumptions and beliefs about life. These are very common and can often cause stress. Do you believe any of these, and if so can you change them? Be honest!
  - I'm a failure if I make a mistake.
  - I should be happy all the time.
  - People must always like me.
  - I must always succeed.
  - Life should be fair.

8. How assertive are you?

Assertiveness is often wrongly confused with being aggressive and self-centred. This could hardly be further from the truth. Assertiveness is about:

- Respect for yourself and others.
- Every human being having equal rights.
- Knowing and expressing your needs.
- Being able to compromise with others.

Everyone's behaviour will vary from situation to situation, but if much of what we do is not assertive, this can cause stress. When we are not assertive, we are likely to be manipulative, aggressive or passively giving in to others.

Here are some suggestions for becoming more assertive if you think that would be useful, but remember to take this slowly, and try out one new thing at a time. If you find these ideas particularly helpful, think about enrolling for a full course, or read up on the subject:

- Saying 'No':
  - Keep it short, and say it confidently and warmly
  - Only give a reason if you want to do so
  - Use a simple phrase you're comfortable with, such as 'I don't want to', or 'I'd rather not'
  - Calmly repeat your 'No' if the first one is not accepted.
- Remember you have these rights:
  - To make a mistake
  - To have your own point of view
  - To fail if you try something
  - To try again
  - To expect others to listen to you.
- Deal with your anger when you're alone by:
  - Punching a pillow, cushion, bed – anything soft that you won't damage
  - Tearing up old newspapers
  - Writing down your angry feelings, then tearing them up!
- Other tips:
  - Value yourself
  - Value other people
  - Work out what you need and want out of life
  - Be prepared to compromise
  - Keep to any point you're making – don't let others distract you from it
  - Keep your voice slow, steady and low-pitched, and stay relaxed
  - Get your feeling of self-worth from within yourself, not just from other people.

9. A problem shared ...

All of us need someone who cares about us and who is interested in what we do. This can bring relief from existing stress, and can even prevent us from feeling stressed in the first place. A problem shared really is a problem halved. Be careful to confide only in those who you can trust, but you can get this important support from a number of places:

- From family/friends/partner

- At work from colleagues (or confidential counselling services provided by some employers)
- From confidential support groups or others in your community.

It is no sign of weakness to seek such support. It can be really effective, and it is a strength to recognize this.

10. Work stress

Stress caused by work is particularly common today. Employers are becoming increasingly aware of this and some are offering training or even counselling to help employees to cope with this. The list of causes would be endless, and most are not easily tackled by the employees themselves, or by those who are self-employed. Long hours, overwork, tight deadlines, and so on, are frequent factors. The most common way to deal with work stress is to cushion yourself from it, using the tips covered so far, especially by relaxation, breaks, social support, a healthy lifestyle, and leisure activities. Think very carefully before you tackle a problem head-on at work. Remember, there may be repercussions for your job or future career.

Here are some other general pointers to think about:

- Are you a square peg in a round hole? Does your personality not really suit the job? If this is the case, and you can change your job, this may be a solution. If you can't, cushioning is the best answer.
- Perhaps you have a low tolerance for stress. Many people do. If so, can you find a less stressful job? If not, cushioning is again the best solution.
- Would learning some new skills make a difference? What about assertiveness, confidence building, time management, team working, delegation or new technology?
- Are courses like this available to you either at work, or from adult education centres?
- Is confidential counselling available at work? Some employers now provide this entirely separate from and independent of the workplace.

Main points

- Can you do anything about the cause?
- Slow down and relax at some point during every day.

- Make sure you are breathing normally.
- Take breaks regularly.
- Adopt a lifestyle that cushions you – regular healthy meals, plenty of sleep, exercise and leisure.
- Gain control of panic attacks.
- Watch out for your thinking causing stress.
- Become more assertive if you need to do so.
- Share your troubles.
- Think about how you can best tackle stress at work.

Useful books and cassettes

Books

A Woman in Your Own Right – Anne Dickson
Assert Yourself – Gael Lindenfield
Assertiveness at Work – Ken and Kate Back
Banish Anxiety – Dr Kenneth Hambly
Beating Stress at Work – Anne Woodham
How to Improve Your Confidence – Dr Kenneth Hambly
How to Stand Up for Yourself – Dr Paul Hauck
I'm OK, You're OK – Thomas Harris
Overcoming Stress – Dr Vernon Coleman
Panic Attacks – Christine Ingham
Self-Help for Your Nerves – Dr Claire Weekes
When I Say 'No' I Feel Guilty – Manuel J. Smith

Audio/video cassettes

A wide range of relaxation aids, music, sounds of nature, etc. is available from:

Matthew Manning, 39 Abbeygate Street, Bury St Edmunds, Suffolk IP33 1LW.
New World Cassettes, Paradise Farm, Westhall, Halesworth, Suffolk IP19 8RH.

Progress Diary

At the end of each week keep a note here of your own rating of how stressed you are on a scale of 0 (no problem) to 5 (maximum problem).

Under the following headings, jot down any actions you've decided to take, and progress on previous new tactics tried etc.:

Date	Stress rating	Actions planned/progress on previous actions

Useful addresses

Here are some useful national addresses and contacts for the GP, some of which may be given to the patient. Information about local branches or services should also be available in local newspapers and directories.

Alcoholics Anonymous, PO Box 1, Stonebow House, Stonebow, York YO1 2NJ.

Alcohol Concern, 275 Gray's Inn Road, London WC1X 8QF.

British Association for Counselling, 1 Regent Place, Rugby, Warwickshire CV21 2PJ.

British Medical Holistic Assocation, 179 Gloucester Place, London NW1 6DX.

Community Education/Adult Education – see local telephone directory.

Depressives Associated, 19 Merley Ways, Wimborne Minster, Dorset BH21 1QN.

Mental Health Foundation, 37 Mortimer Street, London W1N 7RJ.

MIND, National Association for Mental Health. Head Office: Granta House, Broadway, London E15 4BQ.

National Association for Premenstrual Syndrome, PO Box 72, Sevenoaks, Kent TN13 1XQ.

No Panic, 93 Brands Farm Way, Randley, Telford, Shropshire TF3 2JQ.

PAX, 4 Manorbrook, Blackheath, London SE3 9AW.

Relate, National Marriage Guidance, Herbert Gray College, Little Church Street, Rugby CV21 3AP.

Relaxation for Living Trust, 168–170 Oatlands Drive, Weybridge, Surrey KT13 9ET.

Samaritans – see local telephone directory.

Scottish Association for Mental Health, Atlantic House, 38 Gardener's Crescent, Edinburgh EH3 8DQ.

Shelter, 88 Old Street, London EC1V 9HU.

Stresswatch Scotland, 42 Barnweil Road, Kilmarnock KA1 4JF.

Victim Support, Cranmer House, 39 Brixton Road, London SW9 6DZ.

Women's Aid Federation, PO Box 391, Bristol BS99 7WS.

Useful books and cassettes

General books recommended for the General Practitioner

Coping with Stress in the Health Professions – P. Burnard
Counselling and Helping – Stephen Murgatroyd
Life after Stress – Martin Schaffer
Living with Stress – Cary Cooper
Principles and Practice of Stress Managment – Paul Lehrer and Robert
    Woolfolk
Stress – Tom Cox
Stress Management: a Comprehensive Guide – E.A. Charlesworth and
    R.G. Nathan
Stressmanship – Dr Audrey Livingstone Booth
The Skilled Helper – Gerard Egan

Books and cassettes worth recommending to patients

These items are also useful for the GP for background information, and
some are included in the text for the patient booklet.

Books

A Woman in Your Own Right – Anne Dickson
Assert Yourself – Gael Lindenfield
Assertiveness at Work – Ken and Kate Back
Banish Anxiety – Dr Kenneth Hambly
Beating Stress at Work – Anne Woodham
How to Improve Your Confidence – Dr Kenneth Hambly
How to Stand Up for Yourself – Dr Paul Hauck
I'm OK, You're OK – Thomas Harris
Overcoming Stress – Dr Vernon Coleman
Panic Attacks – Christine Ingham

Self-Help for Your Nerves – Dr Claire Weekes
Stress Management: a Comprehensive Guide – E.A. Charlesworth and
    R.G. Nathan
Stressmanship – Dr Audrey Livingstone Booth
Super Confidence – Gael Lindenfield
When I Say 'No' I Feel Guilty – Manuel J. Smith

Audio/video cassettes

A wide range of relaxation aids, music, sounds of nature, etc. is
available from:

Life Foundation School of Therapeutics (UK), Dover Street, Bilston,
    West Midlands WV14 6AL.
Matthew Manning, 39 Abbeygate Street, Bury St Edmunds, Suffolk
    IP33 1LW.
New World Cassettes, Paradise Farm, Westhall, Halesworth, Suffolk
    IP19 8RH.

Appendix 8

Sample page from patient booklet

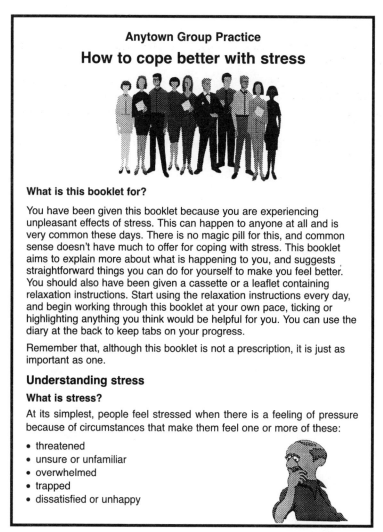

Anytown Group Practice

How to cope better with stress

What is this booklet for?

You have been given this booklet because you are experiencing unpleasant effects of stress. This can happen to anyone at all and is very common these days. There is no magic pill for this, and common sense doesn't have much to offer for coping with stress. This booklet aims to explain more about what is happening to you, and suggests straightforward things you can do for yourself to make you feel better. You should also have been given a cassette or a leaflet containing relaxation instructions. Start using the relaxation instructions every day, and begin working through this booklet at your own pace, ticking or highlighting anything you think would be helpful for you. You can use the diary at the back to keep tabs on your progress.

Remember that, although this booklet is not a prescription, it is just as important as one.

Understanding stress

What is stress?

At its simplest, people feel stressed when there is a feeling of pressure because of circumstances that make them feel one or more of these:

- threatened
- unsure or unfamiliar
- overwhelmed
- trapped
- dissatisfied or unhappy

Figure 1 Sample page from a patient leaflet, including graphics: easily produced using software such as Microsoft Office.

References, bibliography and recommended reading

Alcohol Concern (1995) *Information Pack*. London: Alcohol Concern.

Barlow D.H. (1988) *Anxiety and its Disorders*. New York: Guilford Press.

Beck A.T. (1976) *Cognitive Therapy and Emotional Disorders*. New York: International Universities Press.

Beech H.R., Burns L.E. and Sheffield B.F. (1982) *A Behavioural Approach to the Management of Stress*. Chichester: Wiley.

British Medical Association (1992) *Stress and the Medical Profession*. London: BMA.

Broadhurst P.L. (1958) Determinants of emotionality in the rat: strain differences. *Journal of Comparative Physiological Psychology* **51**: 55–59.

Brow, G. and Harris T. (1978) *Social Origins of Depression*. London: Tavistock.

Cannon W.B. (1929) *Bodily Changes in Pain, Hunger, Fear and Rage*. New York: Appleton.

Carlson C.R. and Hoyle R.H. (1993) Efficacy of abbreviated progressive muscle relaxation training: a quantitative review of behavioral medicine research. *Journal of Consulting and Clinical Psychology* **61**: 1059–1067.

Cooper C., Cooper R.D. and Eaker, L.H. (1988) *Living with Stress*. London: Penguin.

Cooper C.L. and Payne R. (1991) *Personality and Stress: Individual Differences in the Stress Process*. Chichester: Wiley.

Devitt M. (1994) *Review of Staff Support Schemes in Scottish Companies and Organisations*. Edinburgh: Scottish Association for Mental Health.

Ellis A. (1962) *Reason and Emotion in Psychotherapy*. New York: Lyle Stuart.

Ellis A. and Harper R. (1975) *A New Guide to Rational Living*. Los Angeles, CA: Wiltshire.

Eysenck H.J. (1967) *The Biological Basis of Personality*. Springfield, IL: Thomas.

France R. (1993) Effective stress management. In: *Stress Management in General Practice* (Occasional Paper 61). London: Royal College of General Practitioners, 13–17.

France R. and Robson M. (1986) *Behaviour Therapy in Primary Care*. London: Croom Helm.

Friedman M. and Rosenman R. (1974) *Type A Behaviour and Your Heart*. New York: Knopf.

Gelles R.J. (1979) *Family Violence*. Beverly Hills, CA: Sage.

Gersons B. and Carlier I. (1992) Post-traumatic stress disorder: the history of a recent concept. *British Journal of Psychiatry* **161**: 742–748.

Government Statistical Service, (1995), *Criminal Justice – Key Statistics for England and Wales*. London: Government Statistical Service.

Hambly K.N. (1991) *Banish Anxiety*. London: Thorsons/Harper Collins.

Hambly K.N. and Paxton R. (1979) The use of behaviour therapy in general practice. *Update* **19**: 645–648.

Hambly K.N. and Paxton R. (1981) Behaviour therapy in general practice. *The Practitioner* **225**: 1267–1271.

Hardy M. and Heyes S. (1987) *Beginning Psychology*. London: Weidenfeld and Nicolson, 203–205.

Health and Safety Executive (1995) *Stress at Work: a Guide for Employers*. (HS(G) 116). London: HSE.

Holmes T.H. and Rahe R.H. (1967) The social readjustment rating scale. *Journal of Psychosomatic Research* **11**: 213–218.

Howie J.G.R., Hopton J.L., Heaney D.J. and Porter A.M.D. (1992) Attitude to medical care: the organisation of work, and stress among general practitioners. *British Journal of General Practice* **42**: 181–185.

Jacobsen E. (1938) *Progressive Relaxation*. Chicago, IL: University of Chicago.

Jenkins R. (1992) Prevention of mental illness in the workplace. In: Department of Health/Confederation of British Industry, *Prevention of Mental Ill Health at Work*. London: HMSO, 1–23.

Kiecolt-Glaser J.K. and Glaser R. (1991) Stress and immune function in humans. In: Ader R., Felton D.L. and Cohen N., editors, *Psychoneuroimmunology*, 2nd edition. San Diego, CA: Academic Press, 849–864.

Kiely B.G. and McPherson I.G. (1986) Stress self-help packages in primary care: a controlled trial evaluation. *Journal of the Royal College of General Practitioners* **46**: 307–309.

Kobasa S.C. (1979) Stressful life events, personality and health: an inquiry into hardiness. *Journal of Personality and Social Psychology* **37**: 1–11.

Lazarus R.S. (1993) From psychological stress to the emotions: a history of changing outlooks. *Annual Review of Psychology* **44**: 1–21.

Lazarus R.S. and Folkman S. (1984) *Stress, Appraisal and Coping.* New York: Springer.

Lazarus R.S., Deese J. and Osler S.F. (1952) The effects of psychological stress on performance. *Psychological Bulletin* **49**: 293–317.

Lee C. (1995) Telephone hopeline. *Young Scot Magazine* **32**: 26. (Glasgow: *The Herald* in association with the Scottish Community Education Council.).

Lewis B.I. (1959) Hyperventilation syndrome. *California Medicine* **91**: 121–126.

Lum L.C. (1977) Breathing exercises in the treatment of hyperventilation and chronic anxiety states. *Chest, Heart and Stroke Journal* **1**: 7–10.

Mandler G. (1980) The generation of emotion: a psychological theory. In: Plutchik R. and Kellerman H., editors, *Theories of Emotion.* New York: Academic Press. Cited in Hardy M. and Heyes S. (1987) *Beginning Psychology.* London: Weidenfeld and Nicolson, 200–201.

Mason J.W. (1975a) A historical review of the stress field. *Journal of Human Stress* **1** (March): 6–12.

Mason J.W. (1975b) A historical review of the stress field, II. *Journal of Human Stress* **1** (June): 22–35.

Meichenbaum D. (1985) *Stress Inoculation Training.* New York: Plenum.

MIND, National Association for Mental Health (1995) *MIND Information* [booklet]. London: MIND.

Mirrlees-Black C. and Aye Maung N. (1994) *Fear of Crime: Findings from the 1992 British Crime Survey.* (Research Findings, no. 9). London: Home Office Research and Statistics Department.

Muir A.J. (1992) *Step by Step: Self-help for Panic, Anxiety and Phobias.* Kilmarnock: Stresswatch Scotland.

Neighbour R. (1992) *The Inner Consultation.* London: MTP Press.

Nixon, P.G.F. (1989) Human functions and the heart. In: Seedhouse J.

and Cribb A., editors, *Changing Ideas in Health Care*. London: Wiley, 31–65.

Palmer S. (1992) Guidelines and contra-indications for teaching relaxation as a stress management technique. *Journal of the Institute of Health Education* **30/31**: 25–30.

Palmer S. and Dryden W. (1994) Stress management: approaches and interventions. *British Journal of Guidance and Counselling* **22**(1): 5–12.

Pendleton D., Scofield T., Tate P. and Havelock P. (1984) *The Consultation*. Oxford: Oxford University Press.

Romano J.L. (1988) Stress management counselling: from crisis to prevention. *Counselling Psychology Quarterly* **1**: 211–219.

Rotter J.B. (1966) Generalised expectancies for internal versus external control of reinforcement. *Psychological Monographs* **80**: 1–28.

Royal College of General Practitioners. (1993) *Stress Management in General Practice*. (Occasional Paper 61). London: RCGP.

Schaffer M. (1982) *Life After Stress*. London: Plenum.

Seyle H. (1946) The general adaptation syndrome and the diseases of adaptation. *Journal of Clinical Endocrinology* **6**: 117–230.

Seyle H. (1976) *The Stress of Life*. New York: McGraw-Hill.

Seyle H. (1973) The evolution of the stress concept. *American Scientist* **61**: 692–699.

Seyle H. (1974) *Stress Without Distress*. Philadelphia, PA: Lippincott.

Shelter (1995) *Homelessness in England – the Facts* [leaflet]. London: Shelter.

Sterling P. and Eyer J. (1988) Allostasis: a new paradigm to explain arousal pathology. In: Fisher S. and Person J., editors, *Handbook of Life Stress Cognition and Health*. Chichester: Wiley, 635.

Sutherland V.J. and Cooper C.L. (1993) Identifying stress amongst general practitioners: predictors of psychological ill health and job satisfaction. *Social Science and Medicine* **37**: 575–581.

Taylor R. (1992) Case studies in stress. In: Department of Health/Confederation of British Industry. *Prevention of Mental Ill Health at Work*. London: HMSO, 91–102.

Thomson R. (1993) *Mental Illness: the Fundamental Facts*. London: Mental Health Foundation.

Victim Support (1994) *Annual Report*. London: Victim Support.

Walker J. (1995) *The Cost of Communications Breakdown*. Rugby: Relate.

Wheatley D (1991) Stress in women. *Stress Medicine* **7**(2): 73–74.

Wheatley D. (1993) Stress and illness. In: *Stress Management in General Practice*. (Occasional Paper 61). London: Royal College of General Practitioners, 6–11.

Wilkinson G. (1991) Stress: another chimera. *British Medical Journal* **302**: 191–192.

Women's Aid Federation England (1995) *Information Pack*. Bristol: Women's Aid Federation.

Woodham A. (1995) *Beating Stress at Work*. London: Health Education Council.

Worden J.W. (1995) *Grief Counselling and Grief Therapy*. London: Routledge.

Index

Note: references in *italics* indicate figures; there may also be textual references on these pages